RIPLEY'S WORLD

RIPLEY'S WORLD

The Rugby Icon's Ultimate Victory Over Cancer

ANDY RIPLEY

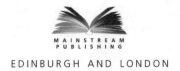

MAINSTREAM
PUBLISHING

EDINBURGH AND LONDON

First published in Great Britain in 2007 by
MAINSTREAM PUBLISHING COMPANY (EDINBURGH) LTD
7 Albany Street
Edinburgh EH1 3UG

ISBN 9781845962944

The author has made every effort to clear all copyright
permissions, but where this has not been possible and
amendments are required, the publisher will be pleased to make
any necessary arrangements at the earliest opportunity.

This book shares the author's experiences of his own prostate
cancer. It should not be construed as medical advice or
as a medical opinion about any other individual's personal
medical condition.

As a matter of policy The Prostate Cancer Charity does
not endorse any products, organisations or the views of
any individuals.

A catalogue record for this book is available
from the British Library

Typeset in Cheltenham and Univers

Printed in Great Britain by
Clays Ltd, St Ives plc

Dare we hope? We dare.
Can we hope? We can.
Should we hope? We must.
We must, because to do otherwise is to waste the most
precious of gifts, given so freely by God to all of us.
So when we do die, it will be with hope and it will be
easy and our hearts will not be broken.

Andy Ripley,
10 June 2007,
Athlone Friary

This book is dedicated to all those in the Club, directly or by proxy,
and to my good friends Steve Muir and Eric Mackie.
THERE ARE NO SHARKS IN KALAMATA BAY

There's nothing worth the wear of winning
But laughter and the love of friends.

Hilaire Belloc

Contents

Foreword

Just as I was starting my rugby-playing career with Leicester Tigers in the late 1970s, Andy's was drawing to a close. Then as now, he was one of the few players who had the respect of everyone connected with the game. When his cancer was diagnosed in 2005, Steve Jones, rugby journalist for the *Sunday Times*, wrote an article in which he said that Andy Ripley was one of the best things to have happened to rugby union. He was right.

We played in one competition together, for the Barbarians; there is a photograph in this book of the team that played in the 1981 Hong Kong Sevens. We were the first and only team from the northern hemisphere to win that particular competition in the twentieth century. It is a fond memory from my playing days.

At the first training session, Andy, who was the captain, said to us, 'Enjoy all of this, guys, because blink and it'll be over.' It seems to me, from a distance, that Andy Ripley has enjoyed life, and I'm glad to say he's still able to blink!

It is a measure of the man that all royalties from this book are to be donated to the Prostate Cancer Charity, and I am delighted to be associated with that cause.

Sir Clive Woodward
July 2007

Introduction

Well, it's Thursday, 25 August 2005, and because I'm totally self-absorbed, self-interested and probably selfish, I've decided to write an account of the past few months of my life and keep a record of those to come.

Why? Because I got up twice last night to go to the lavatory, and my right shoulder doesn't hurt but there is a sort of . . . *awareness*.

Really why? Because two months ago, on Friday, 24 June 2005, at five o'clock in the afternoon, Mr Mike Swinn, consultant urologist at East Surrey Hospital, sat me down in the nurses' room, the only place available, and told me, 'It's unequivocal. You have prostate cancer.'

Nothing too unusual about that: if 32,000 men are diagnosed with prostate cancer in the UK each year, then almost 100 conversations like mine and Mike's take place each day in Britain, and, with about 5 times the population and better detection rates, in the USA some 600 conversations of a similar nature happen each day. There is a slightly larger group of daily conversations with women with breast cancer, and lung cancer comes in at over 100 conversations a day in the UK. Then there is a mass of other dreadful types of mind-boggling, crippling and stultifying illnesses and diseases.

RIPLEY'S WORLD

This isn't about any of them. It's just about me. I told you I was selfish. Written by me and for me.

Andy Ripley
25 August 2005

Part One

It's about five o' clock in the afternoon, and I'm sitting on a chair in the sunshine with my wife and Tim and Maria, who have all come to visit me in East Surrey Hospital. We have sneaked out from Holmwood Ward, Section C, Bed 4, which is on the ground floor, onto a patch of what may one day be grass under two big oak trees, through the door marked 'Strictly No Exit'. We are waiting, just waiting in the sunshine, and it is a wonderful day.

I had been in hospital since the early hours of Sunday, 5 June, so I had got over the initial fretful stage, the stage most new patients seem to experience unless they are too poorly to notice. The stage when you are scared. The stage when you want things to happen now so you can get back home and to your life as it was. The stage before being grateful or really angry. But now, 19 days after having been admitted to East Surrey Hospital, I was pyjama institutionalised and grateful and almost enjoyed the routine and structure in Holmwood Ward, Section C, Bed 4.

'Lighten up, they're all doing their best, this is the best

place to be and, what's more, under the NHS it's free.' This became almost my mantra when talking to new patients. Some of them liked me, some of them didn't. I wanted to be liked. There are eight beds in Holmwood Ward, Section C, and it's the section men get put in after the mixed intensive-care section, Section B. Never found out what they did in Section A. Holmwood is the cardiac ward, and I was put in there initially as it was believed I had had a heart attack in the early morning hours of Sunday, 5 June.

Anyway, if you are an NHS accident and emergency heart patient, you usually get about four days in hospital: one for monitoring, one for an angiogram (a look-see), then up to St George's in London for a stent (a pipe to open up a partially blocked artery) or down to Brighton for a heart bypass, another day back for checking and then into outpatients. I was in for about 20 days; with an average 4-day turnaround per patient, it meant I met about 40 heart patients. No bed was ever empty for longer than a couple of hours.

I know little about medicine, and, apart from an elective clean-up on my knees (a twin arthroscopy in BUPA Gatwick Park), I don't know much about hospitals either. So anything I have to say is purely anecdotal, self-evidently utterly subjective and probably wrong, but it's what I feel or, more precisely, felt at the time.

Even though forty isn't a particularly large sample and East Surrey is just one hospital in a far corner of Surrey, it felt as if the entire world in all its many forms came through the doors, and it was brilliant. I now know that heart attacks can kill you. Whack – you're gone. I now know people can in fact have heart attacks repeatedly and not know, or at least not acknowledge, that they've had one. It's just a pain in the upper left arm or left-hand side of the chest, a bit of breathlessness; it'll get better. It may; without help, it probably won't.

The patients, it seemed to me, had had heart attacks because they were old, it was in the genes, they were fat, smoked, drank too much or were stressed out. No revelations there. However, for me, the big thing in the cardiac ward was that these were often people who had indulged themselves to the point where their health was really suffering, but once they'd realised they weren't going to die, at least probably not today, they were fundamentally happy. The (very) big young (ish) Irish lady would eat and eat all the time, and when her relatives, who resembled a team of marbles on legs, visited, they'd all enjoy themselves and laugh in between handing out the Jaffa Cakes and doughnuts. Compare this to the oncology ward or outpatients, where cancer in its many forms and many stages gradually draws life out of the bodies of its victims. Not much happiness or quick death there, at best a gallows humour and a brave acceptance and resignation.

Still, I'm meandering. How come I was in Holmwood Ward, Section C, Bed 4 which is on the ground floor of East Surrey Hospital at about five o' clock in the afternoon, sitting on a chair in the sunshine with my wife and Tim and Maria, on a patch of warm earth under two big oak trees, waiting in the sunshine?

Friday, 3 June 2005

Well, it all started on Friday, 3 June. Actually, I'd better tell you something about me at this stage, just so that if you want to, you can pigeonhole me. Although, if I am serious about this being written by me, for me, then I should know all about myself already. Do any of us really know ourselves, though? I'll park that one before I wander down too many tributaries all leading nowhere. But does anything lead anywhere? I can be really annoying. I mean, has life just been a process of climbing up a ladder to find eventually you've chosen the wrong wall? Still, enough of this. I guess most of us are fascinated by ourselves and I'm no exception.

But am I in fact writing this because I want it to be read by you? And if so, who are you? Are you me, in the future? Who will then know what happens next? If I survive, this record is redundant. If I die, then working on the basis that everyone's death makes them, for a very short period, a hero, this account may even become commercially viable. You could be a fellow prostate-cancer sufferer looking for clues, for help about your own condition. I'd like that – to be of use to someone else. We all want to make a difference. But, actually, most of all, I'd like to live.

One's own mortality is a strange thing to consider, but with today's awareness in my shoulder, the big question is not just about the quantity of life left but about the quality of that life. It is an academic question at this point in time, but perhaps will not be in the future. For me, if there is no hope and just pain, then, Doctor, bang in the morphine overdose and let me go. The preface to Joseph Oesterling's book *The ABCs of Prostate Cancer*, dated 6 July 1996, movingly details his father's experience:

> After he was diagnosed, not a day went by that my father didn't worry. Living inside the shadow of cancer, he said, was like being trapped inside a cage with a baby lion. In the beginning the lion was small and unthreatening, but he knew that eventually the lion would grow and painfully devour him. Three years after diagnosis, the bone pain began. Then the difficulty urinating. Eventually, the cancer encroached on his spine and my father became paralyzed and bedridden for the last five months of his life.

So, me. I am, as I write in late August 2005, about 57 years and 9 months old, youngest of five children, born in Liverpool, raised in Bristol by my wonderful mum, who left my dad when I was seven. Now living in Surrey with my brilliant family, my wife of 27 years, Elisabeth, and our three children (Mouse, 24, Clouds, 22 and Stef, 19). We've lived in the same house in Dormansland for about 23 years. It's home, we all like it and this summer have all been here together. Mouse (Marcus), after four years of university, can't afford to live anywhere else and is – when he's not, apparently, pimping his ride (whatever that means) – trialling out for London Welsh and being a trainee underwriter; at the time of writing he is in Edinburgh with his girlfriend. Clouds (Claudia) has a holiday job in London before she goes back to her final year at Bath. Stef, this summer, has learned how to cook and will go back to the University of East Anglia for her second year in September. Just another family trying to get by, but it's my family, and it's the best part of my privileged and lucky life.

Friday, 3 June. I'm sitting on the ergometer (a Concept II indoor-rowing machine, in other words, a large hamster's wheel for humans with a clock) at home, doing a low-key session. That's a warm-up on the machine, followed by 6,000 m at a rate of 1 min. 52.5 sec. per 500 m. Including warm-up time, it takes about 22 min. 30 sec. I do, or rather did, something like this on alternate days and rowed on the water about five times a week (Saturday and Sunday morning at about 7.30 in a sweep-crew boat on the Thames at Chiswick and about two or three times on weekdays at 6.30 a.m. in a pair or single scull). All my adult life, I have always enjoyed exercise. Rugby gave me up when I was 41 with broken knees, and then triathlons filled in a gap till 10 years ago I fell in love with rowing. But all my life has been spent running or kicking or hitting a ball or in or on the water. Dull, maybe, but I've loved it.

But on Friday, 3 June, after and during the low-key erg session, I felt a lot more strain than usual – so I took Torben, the dog, for a walk to cool down. My right shoulder ached, same right shoulder that I'm aware of today. I walked about a mile but felt no better, and I was breathless like never before in my life. I turned towards back home, struggling about 25 yards before resting, and then I put the lead on Torben, who didn't know what was happening but somehow pulled me home.

Here's the scary bit: did I go to hospital? Did I call my doctor? No and no. I just took a hot bath and lay down. And, admittedly, I did feel better; but I did nothing. Why is it that men in general (absolutely and in spite of the hormone treatment still including myself in that category) won't get medical advice or help unless it's something very specific, like, say, a broken leg?

Are we lazy? Maybe. Are we stupid? Maybe. Do we just not want to make a fuss? Maybe. Are we frightened to show vulnerability? In the animal kingdom, creatures that show weakness often become somebody else's lunch. Is this the reason? Do we not want to take our clothes off in front of strangers because we men are ashamed of our bodies and particularly our penises? Or can we just not be bothered? Anyway, whatever the reason, I didn't consult anyone.

Saturday, 4 June to Tuesday, 7 June 2005

My shoulder was still painful the next morning, Saturday, 4 June. But I couldn't miss Will and Ness's wedding just because I had a sore shoulder. The wedding was a lot of fun, left the reception in Stockbridge at midnight to the sounds of the Isley Brothers' 'This Old Heart of Mine' –

you can't beat '60s music – and made it home by two. At this stage, the ache in the shoulder was joined by a sharp pain on the left-hand side of my chest, on which a small elephant had also landed. I continued to tell Elisabeth that I was all right, but, luckily, she called NHS Direct, and in the early hours of Sunday morning an ambulance took me to East Surrey Hospital in Redhill. Bless the NHS.

It was a suspected heart attack. They gave me morphine, drips, anticoagulant injections, ECGs, etc. Two days later, there was no more elephant. But it hadn't been a heart attack; it was a pulmonary embolism. Lawks, very early Sunday morning they were still dancing in Stockbridge and I was in intensive care. They caught it early and I got lucky. If it had been left untreated, I could have had my chips. There are 100,000 people a year in the UK who suffer from pulmonary embolisms. 30,000 die. Which is about 10 times the numbers that die annually in road accidents.

From what I can gather (and remember I have no medical training), an embolism is a blood clot that has floated off from somewhere else in the cardiovascular system. The blood in the body has to be pumped by the heart through the lungs to pick up oxygen, so if a blood clot develops in, say, the deep veins of the legs, some of it may go through the heart and then block off part of the lung (pulmonary) circulation, and that blockage in the lungs is a **pulmonary embolism**. Clots are normally dealt with by the body, but some small, medium or large clots under certain circumstances just get dumped in the bloodstream; if a clot is large enough to obstruct the pulmonary circulation, it can lead to collapse or even sudden death without warning.

Why does it happen? Well, anything or any condition that slows down the circulation or makes the blood sticky may lead to pulmonary embolism. So a genetic tendency to clot easily, operations on hips, knee replacements, other major surgery, immobility such as not moving around on long-distance car or plane journeys or bed rest at home or in hospital, pregnancy, advanced cancer and previous deep-vein thrombosis can all be factors leading to pulmonary embolisms.

In half the cases, however, there is no obvious cause. But blood clots are uncommon in healthy people; the body has a very efficient system for dissolving clots. So Dr Sneddon (the heart and embolism specialist at East Surrey), because he is great, he is sort of asking the same question as I'm sort of asking myself. How can I, feeling fine and looking just gorgeous and being the world record-holder for 2,000 m on the indoor-rowing ergometer for the male heavyweight age group 50–60 at a time of 6 min. 7.7 sec. and looking to smash the 60–70 age-group record at 6 min. 23 sec. not be healthy? I've never smoked, drink moderately and am far too vain to have put on weight (117 kg, 6 ft 6 in.).

Dr Sneddon says warfarin and heparin will prevent any further problems while I have a string of tests to find out why I had the embolism. This is Tuesday, my third day in hospital. Scans, injections, venograms, blood samples are taken, and I'm moved from Holmwood Ward, Section B, Bed 1, where everyone is hooked up to oxygen and heart monitors, and into Holmwood Ward, Section C, Bed 4. I should be home by Friday. The treatment for pulmonary embolism is with a tablet called warfarin, but as it takes 48 hours to kick in, a drug called heparin, which thins the blood pretty well instantly, is injected into my stomach (far less dreadful than it sounds) for the first few days. I'm given good advice and plenty of information. I'll need to be regularly monitored to see that the warfarin thins the blood, in my case to between 2 and 3 (1 is the normal-ish INR, or international normalised ratio, level), to prevent further clotting. In six months' time, if Dr Sneddon thinks there are no further risks, I can come off the drug.

There are one million people in the UK taking the anticoagulant warfarin and being monitored. The intention is to find the right balance. The aim is to get the dosage just right so that your blood does not clot as easily as normal, which could possibly result in further embolisms, but it is not so thin as to cause bleeding problems. So, too high an INR and there is a risk of bleeding, either from external cuts or internal injuries; too low, and clotting might come back. Another complication is that warfarin can react with all sorts of other medicines, but the big deal is not only getting the right balance to maximise effect and minimise risk but also, more importantly, you've got to remember to keep taking the tablets, as they say. In hospital, of course, taking the tablets is taken care of. Each day now folds into the next.

Each Day

Hospital is a comforting and comfortable routine which you need to slip into. My routine was as follows: I wake in the morning at about six o'clock and just lie there on the most comfortable bed imaginable, which does just about everything other than boil an egg. Talking of which – 'eggs for breakfast, I'll be bound' – I became constipated, which seems to be the norm in hospitals. I felt like a fraud, as I was surrounded by really poorly people. So, I get up and go to the toilet, and as I have found a pair of really accurate scales, I go and weigh myself, and every morning I am about two pounds lighter than the night before. How do I lose this weight? Where does it go? Two pounds is a bag of sugar – why isn't there a pool of sweat in my bed? Each evening, having eaten only the hospital food, which is good, but keeping off bread and chocolate, I have put back on about a pound in weight. Over ten days, I lose ten pounds, taking no exercise.

After weighing myself, I go back to my bed. At 8.15, Eileen brings us all a cup of tea, and at 8.30 breakfast arrives – just muesli for me. Then the nursing auxiliary comes about 9.00 to take blood pressure and temperature, and about 9.30 they come back and make the bed, and as I can now walk slowly, I go down to the hospital shop and buy a newspaper. What an enjoyable waste of time sudoku is. The doctors make their morning rounds, and then the sister distributes the various medicines. Then maybe there's a scan or an X-ray or another blood test.

If I'm lucky, I speak to the gorgeous young British Asian doctor, Shrilla (who seems to be one of a number of young female Asian doctors who have obviously worked hard at school and medical school – and here am I, the beneficiary), and young Dr Patel, who is destined to be a star and gives me good advice about the potential side effects of having had a pulmonary embolism and taking warfarin. They seem to care for me, but I reckon they care for everyone, and I'm to be discharged once my INR gets over 2; but as I'm 117 kg (or at least was) and in spite of doses in excess of 15 mg, my INR is taking its time to climb. I proudly mention my weight loss to Dr Sneddon; he smiles and says part of it may be due to muscle loss.

Lunch comes at about 1.15, and then it's lights out at 2.00 for a half-hour doze. Eileen back with the tea, visitors and dinner at 6.20, and perhaps the nice lady from Radio Redhill will ask me what request I'd like to hear. Quite frankly, anything other than Bette Midler's 'You Are the Wind Beneath my Wings'. But if I'm going to be judged by the music I choose, a sort of poor man's *Desert Island Discs* for a distant medical corner of Surrey, do I want to go for Van Morrison or Elvis Costello or something by Flotow?

(Pretentious, moi?) The hospital chaplain may call. She's nice and brave, 'cause it seems not everyone is as welcoming as I am. Then the evening medicine round and lights out at about ten. The days merge into each other. I notice that all my original playmates have been replaced and now after ten days I am the old lag. As I mentioned earlier, I am pyjama institutionalised, and I quite like it.

Wednesday, 15 June 2005

It's Wednesday morning, and Dr Sneddon wants a word. All the tests as to why I might have had a pulmonary embolism have shown nothing out of the ordinary. However, the results of a PSA (prostate specific antigen) blood test have come back. For a 57-year-old man, these tests usually give a reading of about 3.5 nanograms per millilitre; mine was out of the ballpark at 133 ng/ml. Not that I noticed, but the world had suddenly changed.

Thursday, 16 June to (eventually) Monday, 20 June 2005

'We can't ignore this.' Over the course of the next two days, I have three digital rectal examinations and am taken off the warfarin; I'm to be kept on the heparin but will be taken off that on Sunday, so that on Monday, 20 June, Dr Raj Kumar can do a prostate biopsy, and I'm to have a nuclear bone scan on the same day. My INR needs to be lower than 1.5, otherwise there is an unnecessary possibility of bleeding during the biopsy operation. Busy.

DREs (Digital Rectal Examinations), what are they? Well, as they say, it does what it says on the tin. They're digital, they're rectal and they're examinations. You lie on the bed on your side with your knees drawn up and the doctor (he/she) will be able to feel your prostate through the rectum wall. This is not dreadful stuff, well, leastwise not for the examinee, and I'm sure the examiner has heard all there is to hear about putting your finger up people's asses for a livelihood. That is the crucial word: livelihood. It's your life they may be saving. Well, actually and more specifically, it's my life they may be saving.

I reckon the doctors/urologists/oncologists have a good idea of what they are looking for, and they seem to set a lot of store by the DRE, which is primarily a feel of the back of the wall of the prostate gland, the front not being readily accessible. All three, Shrilla the ward doctor, Dr Kumar the urologist and, the following day, Mr Swinn the consultant, said pretty much the same thing. My prostate wasn't unusually large for a man of my age, but it was slightly distended on the right-hand side. I learn later that 20 cubic centimetres is the usual volume of the prostate. Quite frankly, I don't know the size of something with a volume of 20 cc, but the standard size comparison seems to be a walnut for a young man and an orange for a man on a bus pass.

I was reading *Life of Pi*, and Dr Kumar told me that although he really liked the book, as a Muslim from Bombay, he'd noticed a number of annoying inaccuracies in locations and names, which for him spoiled some of the enjoyment. He also told me that if the prostate is enlarged and hard, like when you feel your forehead with your finger, this isn't as good as if it's soft, like the skin on the end of your nose.

Following the DRE, Mr Swinn wanted to get the result of Monday's **biopsy operation** before deciding what, if anything, should be done. He was at pains to point out that there was a small risk of infection, as the probe had to go through the rectum wall, as well as a possibility of incontinence and of bleeding in both semen and urine after the operation, although these should be short-term problems. The operation would last ten minutes and I would be given a small local anaesthetic and a course of antibiotics. I think there must be some sort of NHS ruling that doctors are obliged to tell patients all the potential side effects of operations and medicines. I suppose this is a good thing, and presumably it's done so patients are prepared for the worst. Maybe it's also done because patients and doctors and hospitals are living in an increasingly litigious culture. If you happen to be amongst the unlucky, say, 5 per cent that picks up a possible but unlikely side effect of some operation, maybe it is good to have been made aware it might happen, and maybe the hospital has to protect itself, does need a bit of paper signed by you. However, it also has the effect of raising an already high anxiety level.

So I'm off the warfarin and back into the comfort of the ward routine. I should mention that at this stage I had no **symptoms of prostate cancer**. These are normally written up as abnormally short intervals between passing urine, particularly being woken up in the night by the need to pass urine and/or being unable to hold on after feeling the need to pass urine, and/or a poor stream, hesitancy, terminal dribbling or incomplete emptying, and/or pain while urinating or passing blood in the urine. I should add that if you do have any of these, it's far more likely to be a benign prostatic hyperplasia (BPH) than prostate cancer.

However, I had none of these symptoms, nor was I in any pain. In fact, now my pulmonary embolism appeared to be breaking down, I was feeling great. People around me were very ill and two patients died on the ward. June in 2005 was a warm, sunny month. I sat and sunbathed on the patch of earth outside the back entrance to Holmwood Ward and started to go for walks across the nearby golf course and onto the North Downs Way. It was glorious. Friends and family who visited me got a two-mile trek over the Surrey hills.

However, I couldn't help noticing the staff and doctors were particularly kind to me. I thought, well, this is because I'm such a great bloke; then it crossed my mind that maybe they knew something I didn't. Well, they knew I had a PSA score of 133, had had three DREs in quick succession and was being rushed into a biopsy and bone scan in double-quick time.

I didn't realise it at the time, because I didn't know much about it, but my 133 PSA score was what was defining me. Because I knew so little, I began to read stuff. Periodically, in between weighing myself and walking on the North Downs Way, I'd sneak out of Holmwood Ward, Section C, Bed 4. In East Surrey Hospital in the canteen on the second floor, there is an Internet connection, and I went and found out about the **PSA test**.

First, there is a question, and that question is almost the same one raised by Mr Swinn detailing to me all the possible side effects of a biopsy, which took me from a benign state of ignorance to a state of raised concern: do men really want to know about the potential side effects of a biopsy? Well, the answer is, it depends. But on balance, for me, better to know before the operation, deal with the possibility but don't bother crossing Anxiety Bridge. So it's also understandable to pose the question, do men want to know whether they do or do not have prostate cancer? Well, this is a no-brainer. Of course they want to know, because maybe something can be done about it, and then maybe you don't get to die.

The PSA test is used by doctors as an aid to detecting prostate cancer. It measures the level of prostate specific antigen in the blood, and a raised level of this substance can indicate prostate cancer. I had noticed that in all the charts and gradings and stages of prostate cancer, along the X axis, the PSA level, there were various bands, like 0–2, 2–4, 4–7, 7–10, 10–20, and then, on the far right-hand side, greater than 20. At 133, my score would seem to be six times greater than the outer reaches of statistical significance. No wonder this number defined me; no wonder everyone was so nice as I bounded around on those sun-blessed June days. Experience had taught them that 133 might well mean the cancer has spread out of the capsule into the local tissue and into the bones and, to use the new word I'd learned, metastasised to who knows where. But I felt good: no pain and no symptoms.

Monday, 20 June. The biopsy was scheduled for 12.30 (outpatients were always given the morning appointments). I was to go through the usual morning hospital routine, with a blood test to check that the effects of the warfarin and heparin had worn off, then I was scheduled for a bone scan at two o'clock.

So I take myself down to the oncology department reception and am shown into Dr Kumar's office. Hille, the Swedish nurse, checks the details and phones to check my INR reading; the number comes back 1.6. This is too high to operate, as there is a danger of bleeding. Mike Swinn pops his head round the door, no reason to take the bleed risk, do it on Wednesday. Hille walks me back to Holmwood, tells the duty sister, who says no, my INR reading this morning was 1.2, not 1.6. Check on the computer, the duty sister is right. Dr Kumar and Hille give up their lunch hour to do the biopsy. It's their seventh of the morning.

For the **trans-rectal ultrasound biopsy (TRUS biopsy)** you get in the same position as for the DRE. I was given a local anaesthetic, I lay on my side and Hille let me hold her hand. Maybe it is undignified, but at no stage did I feel any indignity, just a sense that kind, professional people were doing their job. It's not a dissimilar level, although a different type, of discomfort as you might experience visiting the dentist, say. A needle is inserted through your rectum wall into the prostate and samples are taken. There is a sort of twang, like an air pump, but I felt nothing. Usually eight, sometimes ten samples are taken, but I had twelve. I think, as I would be going back on anticoagulants, they wanted to nail it first time. Back to Section C, Bed 4. I lay down; Eileen had kept my lunch.

At 1.55, in preparation for the **bone scan**, I walked down to the nuclear medicine department, and they injected me (most injections or blood samples were in the vein in the inside of the arm) with a small amount of radioactive substance. I went back to Bed 4 and drank lots of water, then, about three hours later, I went back for the bone scan. If there are active cancer cells in the bones, they take up the radioactive substance and this is shown on the scanner. The actual scanning process takes about half an hour. The bone scan is totally painless – you just lie there – but it scared me, because this is not a specific test for cancer and uptake can be due to other conditions, such as old healed fractures, benign diseases of the bone or arthritis. Twenty years of contact sport had left me with lots of healed fractures, and I had been told following an X-ray five years earlier that I had arthritis in both my shoulders. If there were to be an abnormality, how could they determine what was causing it? The results would take five to ten days to come back.

Tuesday, 21 June to Thursday, 23 June 2005

The next few days are fine, the sun is shining, and I'm feeling good and determined to deal with stuff only if and when it arises. After the biopsy for two days, particularly in the morning, I pass blood. For a man, it is a strange sensation, not physically but visually, to pass blood-tinged urine. But it's Beaujolais Nouveau red, not Scarlett O'Hara. Within three days, the urine is clear, the walking has cleaned out my bowels without any medication, there is no infection from the biopsy and I'm back on huge doses of warfarin (18 mg) and heparin to thin my blood. The hospital routine is still comfortable and comforting. The 21st of June is the summer solstice. The sun is at right angles to the tropic of Cancer, and, for those who are into that sort of stuff, we have just moved into the fourth zodiacal constellation, between Gemini and Leo: Cancer.

Friday, 24 June 2005

So we are back to where we started. It's about five o' clock in the afternoon, and I'm sitting on a chair in the sunshine with my wife and Tim and Maria, who have all come to visit me in East Surrey Hospital. We have sneaked out from Holmwood Ward, Section C, Bed 4, which is on the ground floor, onto a patch of what may one day be grass under two big oak trees, through the door marked 'Strictly No Exit'. Waiting in the sunshine.

Mr Swinn walks over to me and says he has a verbal report about the biopsy, would I like to come and talk to him, and would my wife like to come with me. I don't know why, but I want to see him by myself.

Mr Swinn is immediate and direct. Next week he is at a conference in Scotland and the fortnight afterwards he is on holiday, but he wanted to speak to me before he left. He has only a verbal report from the pathologist; the written report will come later. However, based on the pathologist's verbal report, 'It's unequivocal. You have prostate cancer.'

'Unequivocal' is an angular, direct word with no softness. I have prostate cancer. Mike adds 'middling prostate cancer'. He knows I had a PSA of 133. For me, this isn't in the script, but I feel actually quite strong. He then says that the cancer is probably beyond surgery. There is a possibility, maybe, of radiotherapy, but if the cancer has spread outside the prostate, they will need to find out how far. There is little point in surgery or radiotherapy if there is no possibility of a cure, as each of these methods of treatment have side effects. He is recommending putting me on hormone treatment, but I should understand this is not a cure, although it can reduce prostate cancer and should slow both its spread and the speed of its progression. As with all treatments, however, there are side effects.

I found myself suddenly asking almost banal questions, which even to me at the time sounded like some B-movie script, like, 'How long have I got Doc?' Well, poor old Mr Swinn. As I found out later, he'd just spent six hours in surgery removing someone's bowel, it was now late Friday afternoon, and I imagine he had issues in his life, like all of us. He probably wanted to get home and watch *The Simpsons*, and here he was being asked a question to which he really had no answer, not with any certainty. I mean, how long is a piece of string? But he was never less than professional, not wanting to give false hope, not wanting to make me cross Anxiety Bridge. I felt quite warm towards him. He'd been the messenger before and will be for the rest of his working life. He stayed with me. I asked him if I could go and speak with my wife. I went outside to Elisabeth and Tim and Maria. Maria had nine years before been diagnosed with breast cancer and had made a full recovery. I told them what Mr Swinn had said. Tim and Maria were great – what a thing to dump on a mate, but I suppose that's what mates are for. They left Elisabeth and myself together under the oak tree on a patch of earth in the evening sunshine.

Now, my wife is rubbish when it comes to me walking into the house on a wet muddy day after taking the dog for a walk just after she has done the hoovering and me forgetting to take my shoes off. 'Well, they're not that dirty' doesn't work. She goes nuts, and quite frankly I'd do the same if I'd just done the hoovering. However, although when it comes to the little stuff (*this is not little stuff*), quite rightly, she spits and kicks and has done since the day we got married in her home village, Seefeld in Austria, on 22 January 1977, at the other stuff, the big stuff, she is brilliant. The eldest of five children, when she was 17, her dad, who was a plumber, died of bowel cancer aged 49. Her mum died of breast cancer aged 61. Elisabeth is OK. We are OK. I can't begin to imagine what it is like for those men diagnosed without the support of a family. A Macmillan nurse was on hand, but Elisabeth and I were lucky. We had each other and that was enough and we didn't need the Macmillan nurses' offered kind services. Mike organised everything and the matron arranged for further heparin shots and for me to pick up my medication the following morning. I could go home.

We drove home through the country lanes, over the M23, and pulled in by the side of the road. Were we really OK with this? Yeah, we'd handle it. The hard part was about to come: how do we tell the kidlets? Do we say anything? Stef was at home and Mouse would be there when we got back and Clouds would be there an hour later. We decided to say nothing until they were all together, and then I'd tell them, together.

I was feeling surprisingly good and strong. Was I in complete denial? Or was I just happy to be out of hospital? I almost felt empowered. I'd also recovered from a pulmonary embolism and, by accident, had had the prostate cancer in my body identified. I was sort of lucky. I'd spent about three weeks with good and kind people, staff and patients. Stef and Mouse were happy to see me back home and when Clouds arrived on that sunny 24 June evening, in the front room I told them how it was, at least as far as I knew. Somehow I felt I was letting them down. We had a family hug, tears were spent. 'Cancer' is such an emotive word.

Having told my family, I thought for a while about what I should do next. Should I do anything? I phoned my brother and sisters; we have always been a close family. Then, that evening, I decided to send an email to my friends. Why? It wasn't so much sharing a burden as self-preservation, in that I didn't want to repeat the same fairly unreal conversation. I've reproduced that first email I sent out below.

> Many apologies for this email as although I've done a bit of gardening on it, it is my email contact list and includes many types of relationships, so some may be wondering why they've received it, and to others who deserve far more than something that has the appearance of a Christmas round robin, please forgive me.
>
> Quick update: Friday, 3 June, did an easy ergo session (6,000 m at a steady 1 min. 52.5 sec., takes 22 min. 30 sec.). Felt unusually bad – so took the dog for an ease-off walk, as my right shoulder was hurting, got about a mile and nothing was easing off, breathless

– Torben pulled me home. Being of the Monty Python school of medicine – 'It's only a scratch' – took a hot bath and lay down – felt better.

Still sore the following Saturday morning, Will and Ness's wedding, which was great, drove back home from Stockbridge at midnight, got home at 02.00. At which point the ache in the shoulder was joined by a sharp pain on the left-hand side of my chest and a small elephant. Still told Elisabeth it was OK – fortunately for me she called NHS Direct, an ambulance took me to East Surrey Hospital – suspected heart attack, morphine, drips, anticoagulant injections, ECGs, etc. Two days later, the elephant had gone, it wasn't a heart attack but a pulmonary embolism. Got it early, got lucky. Untreated, it could have been an early exit.

Warfarin and heparin would sort it out. Then had a whole series of tests to find out why I'd had clots on the lung. Scans, injections, blood samples – nothing out of the ordinary other than a PSA (prostate specific test). These tests usually are about 3.5 ng/ml, mine was in the stratosphere at 133. Lots of clinical tests and then off the anticoagulants, so that last Monday they could do a prostate biopsy and a nuclear bone scan. Still in hospital, getting sort of pyjama institutionalised, the NHS is brilliant. Back on warfarin, got the results this weekend.

Although have not had the bone scan or a written report, verbally it seems I have got middling prostate cancer. An MRI scan and the bone scan will give some indication if it has broken out of the prostate and into other parts of the body. I'm being given hormone treatment, starting tomorrow, which hopefully will have the effect of reducing the PSA. There are side effects, impotence and tiredness, but if the PSA drops then although it will not cure, it will delay, defer the spread. Downside: could already be too invasive and/ or in spite of the hormone treatment, things may move rapidly. Upside: the scans will show it is contained and there will be some value in radiotherapy, which can be a cure and not just a delay of uncertain tenor.

At home with my wonderful family, surprisingly feeling good and strong, am happy to let people know everything, will even get back on the erg tomorrow. I've been just blown away by two things: how lucky I've been not to have fallen to the pulmonary embolism and to still be here with the help of the NHS; and secondly how wonderful everybody has been – I feel really loved. I intend to be and do exactly as you would hope and expect, and will continue to lead as normal a life as possible for as long as possible. You may wish to phone or email but really there is nothing else to say and you're gonna get another update sometime, but if you like you can send me a get-well card!

Lots of love, Andy

24 June 2005

I'm sure that of the 100 men who today in the UK will be told they have prostate cancer, like me, many will find that if there is a silver lining to this disease, it's the love and support of friends and family, which have given and give me strength. I know some people may wish to be private, to keep things to themselves, not to burden others. I can only admire and respect their privacy. For me, it was the letters, cards and emails from people who said kind things because they felt they might not get another chance that gave me joy.

Saturday, 25 June to Monday, 27 June 2005

The next couple of days were anxious, but it was sunny and I was not in pain. I was still going to the hospital each morning for a heparin injection until the warfarin kicked in and to take my INR to over 2.00. I liked going back to Holmwood Ward. On the Saturday morning, I was given the tablets to start the **hormone treatment**. So on Saturday, 25 June, I began my 30-day oral course of Casodex 50 mg (bicalutamide), an anti-androgen, and on 7 July, I had my first injection of Zoladex 3.6 mg (goserelin), a luteinising hormone-releasing hormone (LHRH). This, for me, was by injection in the stomach, given by Lynne, the nurse at Lingfield Surgery, who was also checking my INR level. The injection is OK, but, me being a big wuss, Lynne gave me a very small local anaesthetic.

The reason hormone therapy was probably the appropriate treatment for me was that, with a PSA of 133 and a pathologist's report on my biopsy giving me a Gleason score of 7 (the Gleason grade rates the likely aggressiveness of a cancer on a scale of 2–10), it was likely I had locally advanced cancer that might already have spread.

It seems to me, with my little knowledge, that the methods of treating the many cancers come down to three options: surgery, radiotherapy and controlled poison. Which one, if any? Or in what combination? Which one is appropriate will depend on the type and stage of the cancer and the age and well-being of the patient. Each one of these options comes with side effects, and if the cancer is beyond the reach of these current options, there seems little point in surgery or radiotherapy and their associated side effects.

Hormone treatment comes under the category of poison. (Chemotherapy is another poison that can extend the runway of life a bit further but also comes with its own brand of side effects.) It is not a cure, but it may limit and/or defer the spread of the cancer. It can also be used in conjunction with radiotherapy or, although this is less likely, surgery. For me, it was the way to go while the hospital checked how far the cancer had spread, via MRI scans, nuclear bone scans and CT scans, and determined whether or not there was any point in going through the hassle of radiotherapy. Surgery, for me at my stage, was a non-starter.

Low-dose Casodex (50 mg) blocks the action of testosterone in the body. Testosterone is the agent of growth and spread of prostate cancer, so this treatment, hopefully, inhibits the spread of the disease. There are a whole series of types of anti-androgens, each with their own characteristics. I don't intend to detail these, since I'm not qualified and others have already covered the ground. In the UK, the current industry standard text seems to be *The Prostate: Small Gland, Big Problem* by Professor Roger Kirby.

LHRH analogues such as Zoladex block testosterone production, which appears to be the chemical equivalent/ alternative to the surgical procedure of removing the testicles (**orchidectomy**). Castration seems a brutal option but apparently has an immediate short-term effect and, like Zoladex, can decrease and/or delay the spread of cancer.

How long is that bit of string? It depends. It depends where you start from, but the figure bandied about seems to be 18–36 months. However, most of the doctors I've seen do talk about some patients having much longer deferrals of the spread. I'm also sure there are some patients who aren't talked about for whom the poison is less effective ultimately. Although the poison kills hormone-sensitive cells, eventually these cells are replaced by hormone-insensitive cells, which do not respond to the treatment.

Anyway, the major short-term side effects of taking Zoladex with an anti-androgen are listed as a loss of sex drive and impotence. At this early stage, I had no side effects. Although three weeks in hospital, a pulmonary embolism and being diagnosed with locally advanced prostate cancer doesn't do too much for your libido. We did have sex once during this period, and as I was still getting erections, I suppose we could have had a reasonable sex life, as we had had before 4 June 2005. However, besides a loss of libido, probably accentuated by the sight of blood in my semen after the biopsy, I also had the thought that if the agent of change was testosterone, then wasn't it better not to produce the stuff? Again, most doctors I spoke to suggested this was absolutely not the case, but it was my body and that's how I felt. However, the most important conversations I had were with Elisabeth, who was massively kind, sensitive and thoughtful – *for better, for worse* never seemed more appropriate.

An article in the *British Journal of Urology International* entitled 'Sexual, Psychological and Dyadic Qualities of the Prostate Cancer "Couple"' indicates that erectile dysfunction (impotence) is the commonest complication and long-term side effect of prostate-cancer treatment. It is often the side effect that the patient worries about most. In a sample of 103 men with prostate cancer and their partners, it was found that patients generally rated their own sexual performance and satisfaction lower than their partners rated theirs and were inaccurate about how they were perceived by their partners.

At the time I'm writing this, today, 1 September 2005, I'm still in limbo land as regards any certainty as to whether I am still potent. Self-evidently, if you have your testicles removed, impotence is a certainty and non-reversible. If you are on Zoladex, it seems from what I've read, you/I will become impotent, which appears to me to be chemical castration. This may not be permanent if you stop taking the drug. However, stop taking the drug, and you have not been cured and the cancer will presumably come back. I'll let you know as time unfurls. If you keep taking Zoladex over time, as this is a poison, there are other side effects: bone thinning, diabetes and liver damage are some of the contenders mentioned. Physical castration or chemical castration, each obviously comes with its own set of concerns. Not a great choice, really, but for most men, although possibly not all, better than dying.

Actually, I should mention it here, I have no real idea what way this will all go, but I don't intend rewriting anything in this account as time does unfurl and I gain the benefit of hindsight. I'll keep this record like a diary, just write about what I feel and what I know at the time of writing, even though events in the future may overwhelm, for better or worse, those concerns and feelings I have at a given moment in time.

I also know, assuming the worst, that as my quantity of life looks increasingly limited as future information is unfurled in a way that confirms my and the doctors' potential fears, there is absolutely no point in worrying about that particular concern, as the limited time I have left should be enjoyed and not wasted in worrying about dying. I don't know the word, but if remorse (which I've always considered the most pointless of emotions) is wasting time agonising over what has been, over something you can never change, then the obverse of remorse must be wasting time worrying about what may never be. Even if it does happen, think about the time wasted in agonising about it. I seemed to have developed in my head this idea of not crossing Anxiety Bridge.

The one big difference, though, is that whereas you certainly can't change the past, you can maybe change the future. Hope has to be the beacon, and where there's life there's hope. My great-grandmother on my father's side, born in York in 1864, was the fourth child of Mary Hasling, an Irish immigrant who married Zachariah Waite. Actually, my paternal great-grandmother was not their fourth but their thirteenth child. Nine had died in childbirth and she was apparently going the same way, but, according to family history, Zachariah said, 'Where there is life there is hope.' She lived and was called Hope Waite and lived a fine life until 1930 and is buried in Thimbleby Churchyard in Lincolnshire.

Tuesday, 28 June 2005

Quite a lot of time at this stage was spent waiting for the next result of a PSA test (which could be an acronym for permanent state of angst) or bone scan or whatever. I've reproduced below my second email sent on 28 June.

> Thank you so much for your kindness and love and cards and calls. Well, kids, thanks to you it's working, the results of the nuclear bone scan were that I'm clean, no bone cancer.
>
> I've still got a PSA of 133 but maybe that's just a number, perhaps the cancer has seeped a bit locally and there may be knockbacks and the MRI scan next week will show what we have to deal with, but I'm taking the hormone tablets and feeling good and maybe, just maybe, it is contained in the prostate.
>
> I feel there is a really good and genuine chance not only to extend the runway, but get cured.
>
> Love Andy
>
> The glorious 28th June 2005.

The Macmillan nurse at East Surrey Hospital had phoned me and given me the news. I asked her if this changed anything. She said, yes, it's really good news. You should also come into the hospital outpatients on 14 July to meet Dr Julian Money-Kyrle, the oncology consultant, who will have all your scans and tests and the written report on the biopsy from the pathologist. On 7 July, Lynne gave me my first Zoladex injection.

Friday, 8 July 2005

Some of you may recall that on 7 July 2005 four young British men felt that by killing themselves and more than fifty innocent victims and maiming another two hundred they would make the world a better place. Work that one out and stay fashionable. As a result of this, rather than using the train, which wasn't running, at about six o'clock in the evening I was driving my motorbike, with Clouds as pillion, on the A23 through Brixton on my way home. Stuff happens, a lady car driver pulls out of a side street, I see her, and she then sees me. Too late. I lay the bike down and bounce along the road. Inside my crash helmet, I'm thinking, as my last INR count was 3.6, am I going to get internal bleeding in my head? I stop bouncing. Clouds is OK. The bike is bleeding oil and water and looking a bit the worse for wear. The lady car driver is OK. Some kind people pick me and the bike up. Slightly shocked, as is Clouds, but I don't seem to be bleeding, at least not on the outside. Glad I bought decent boots, gloves, helmet and jacket.

We swap addresses, and I notice the lady works for the NHS and her Christian name is Comfort.

The bike is a Triumph Rocket. I'd bought it about a year before and driven about 5,000 miles on it. The accident was a bit like my first motorbike prang. When I was 16, in 1964, I'd bought a Bantam 125 for £19. We lived in Bristol, and somehow I'd managed to drive it from the motorcycle shop in Westbury on Trym four miles home to Belvedere Road, Redland, without a helmet and, miraculously, without mishap. Then, in the full flush of youthful pride and ownership, I drove it to the end of Belvedere Road and straight into a car – entirely my fault. The very kind car driver took me home and told my mum if I was going to ride a motorbike I should at least learn how to drive. He then gave me the telephone number of the RAC/ACU motorcycle course, which I signed up for. I never saw him again, but I reckon he probably saved my life. I've been driving bikes on and off ever since. The big difference is that you don't bounce so well at 57 as you do at 16.

Standing by the road in Brixton, wanting to be pretty much anywhere else, I then discover that the engine turns over. It's stuck in second gear, but with a big engine that's OK. I drive home slowly. My back starts to hurt. About five days later, when I am having an MRI spine scan, the very nice nurse tells me I've cracked two ribs back left and one front right. When I get home, Elisabeth isn't too happy. Not surprising – this hasn't been a great month for me, but it hasn't been a barrel of laughs for her either. I put the bike in the garage and then realise the pain in my chest is not dissimilar to the pain I felt on 4 June when I had the pulmonary embolism. The big difference is that now when I lie still, provided I don't breathe deeply, laugh or move, the pain goes. Playing rugby, I've bust a few ribs and, as painfully, done something to the intercostal muscles. I recognise the pain. Most importantly, I don't have a headache and I've no external bleeding. I reckon the best thing to do is lie still for a few days in front of the TV and watch the Tour de France.

What I found strange was that whereas I had previously wanted to see people, now I couldn't really move, I didn't want to see anyone. I was in pain and thought they'd think it was the embolism or the cancer; I didn't want to look badly winged. Three days, and the pain began to ease off.

There I was, a walking pharmacy, full of warfarin, heparin, Casodex and Zoladex, but I couldn't bring myself to take painkillers. I saw Lynne for my INR check-up on Monday, 11 July, she made me see the blessed Dr Gardener, we had a little chat and he definitely raised his eyebrows re riding a motorbike on warfarin. I was due to see the oncologist on 14 July at East Surrey Hospital.

I really liked watching the Tour de France on TV. To date, I have received five copies of *It's Not About the Bike*. Sure, Lance isn't a cuddly hero (he's more like the word 'unequivocal' – angular), but ever since – was it in the fifth tour he won? – he took that dramatic detour across a field to avoid a fallen rider, he, in my eyes, has been heroic. The cancer stuff – well, he got lucky and dealt with it.

Thursday, 14 July 2005

Elisabeth and I drove to East Surrey Hospital for my appointment with Dr Julian Money-Kyrle. The ribs apart, I was feeling good. Each oncology ward must have its own feel but I'm sure there's a universal characteristic: people look brave but not good. The news is going to be OK or really bad; cancer deals in absolutes. I don't know what the private medicine suite is like, but I was very much in the hands of the NHS and happy to be so.

Julian had a bow tie, and I felt we would have had a bit of a laugh together in different circumstances. Neither of us was laughing at 2.30 on 14 July. He confirmed the original PSA reading of 133 told to me on 15 June; the blood test must have been taken a couple of days before. He confirmed the results of the bone scan were negative and the Gleason score of 7 from the biopsy done on 20 June. He let me know that on the basis of the MRI scan it was likely I had locally advanced prostate cancer, which might have seeped into the adjacent glands on the right-hand side, the seminal vesicles and maybe some of the lymph nodes and possibly other areas in the pelvis. He gave me a look at the MRI scan, which showed layered cross sections of the pelvis. The prostate gland looked distended, but it was not readily apparent to me that there was any dilation of the nodes, and even if there was, was it necessarily cancerous or could it just be due to the fact I had had an arthroscopy on my right knee that had got badly infected? The recent phlebitis attack on my right thigh could also have caused a reaction. I didn't know, but it struck me that Julian wasn't absolutely certain either. I assume that unless you get the cells out and probably under a microscope, nothing is certain. However, experience must also play a big part, and the markers are the DRE, the PSA, the pathologist's biopsy report and the various scans. But this cancer stuff dictates that although there are scientific bits, it is an art. Why? Because there is so much uncertainty. Because, I reckon (without any medical knowledge), any cancer has the ability to change its characteristics at any time. The certainty, the value, the shape today need not be the same tomorrow. Each cancer cell will have its own characteristics and will change and mutate according to those characteristics.

Julian confirmed that the hormone therapy was at present the most appropriate treatment, that surgery was not to be recommended, as this might not resolve the problem but could generate various side effects. However, he then said that the Royal Marsden, the specialist cancer hospital in London, had agreed to take me if I was willing to be a test candidate, as they were testing a new form of radiotherapy called IMRT (intensity modulated radiotherapy) and this form of treatment might be appropriate in my case. I was willing.

Julian then told me that the Marsden needed two further scans, which were to be done in East Surrey Hospital in the next couple of weeks: a nuclear bone scan and an MRI spine scan. Also, although I'd recently had a biopsy, the hormone treatment had only just started and it was about three weeks since my first PSA test, I was to have another one that day. The Marsden would be in touch with me to arrange an appointment.

I felt that, whatever the outcome, they were doing their best for me. I wrote another email after seeing the oncologist, as detailed below:

> Could have got wiped by the pulmonary embolism on 4 June; thanks to my wife calling NHS Direct and them being fab – didn't.
>
> Could have got wiped by the motorbike crash on 8 July – didn't. Ribs still sore but will soon be frisky as a flea.
>
> Bastille Day, 14 July, just seen the oncologist, who has got all my results, biopsy, bone scans, MRI scans, pathology reports, etc. Well, it seems I'm just on the edge, but if I hadn't had a PSA test because of the blood clot I would have continued in my blissful ignorance until just extending the runway and pain reduction would have been all that could have been of any value. The cancer is on one side of the prostate and does appear to have seeped out into some of the adjacent lymph nodes, but it is not in the bones. Surgery may resolve the prostate cell growth but wouldn't address the seepage. So that's not a viable option. Gleason score, for those who know about this stuff – 7. High but not 10.
>
> So just taking the hormone treatment (which I've been on for three weeks) is not a cure but has the opposite effect of anabolic steroids, it limits testosterone, which is the prostate cancer's agent, and inhibits for a period (six months, one year, ten

years – who knows) any further cancer growth and should reduce the PSA score. Side effects while taking the drug: impotence and muscle loss, possible hot flushes and generally getting in touch with your feminine side. Can't wait.

However the doctor, bless him, suggested I could take a particular type of radiotherapy course which is only available at the Marsden, which is still in the development stage, something to do with varying the strength of the radiotherapy dose. It could offer a complete cure. There are potential side effects, like frying bits of you you don't really want fried.

Anyway, I'm feeling great and I now have a chance of getting away with this. I won't send any more emails out 'cause everyone has got their own concerns and I'm sure you don't want to hear about the minutiae of my ups and downs. Thank you for your kind thoughts and letters and emails, if I haven't replied, forgive me. They meant and mean a lot to me.

Lots of love (see, the hormone tablets are already spinning their magic),

Andy

Friday, 15 July to Tuesday, 16 August 2005

I have the MRI spine scan on 27 July and the nuclear bone scan on 8 August and the Marsden, good as their word, make an appointment at their site in Sutton, Surrey, for 2.30 on 17 August. My 14 July PSA has fallen from 133 to 95 – not huge but OK under the circumstances and in the right direction. My ribs start to feel better, but I can't move too well, cough, laugh or breathe deeply until the end of July.

Still taking the warfarin, but to keep in the 2–3 INR range, the daily dose is 12 mg. Have my second Zoladex injection on 4 August. Still getting erections, but as I feel ejaculating would only kick up my testosterone, I don't bother. My testicles do appear to be shrinking. Am I bothered? Sure, I am, but in my head is the view, right or wrong, that this is only a temporary state of affairs.

August is a good month. As my ribs improve, I can start walking and exercising again. Every day, I feel better. I even manage to go rowing again. About once a week, on Wednesdays, I row on Bewl Bridge Reservoir in a coxed four with the guys who taught me to row ten years previously. We are almost an adaptive four: the cox, Margaret, is a chronic asthmatic, and her heart is on the right-hand side of her body; Lawrence, aged 55, has dizzy spells; I've just had a pulmonary embolism, broken three ribs and been diagnosed with cancer; John, 69, has just been told he has Parkinson's disease; and Mike, 53, sadly for him, is a doctor. Hugh, 62, who steps in when one of us can't make it, seems fine. We go out once a week and afterwards eat buns and talk about stuff. My weight since leaving the hospital has gone up from 107 kg to 114 kg.

Life goes on well, and I am learning to adapt to my new status, whatever that is. On Saturdays, I go and row at Tideway Scullers School (TSS), either in a pair or a coxless four. What is strange is that at TSS, early 2005, about late March, after a Saturday morning outing (7.30 to about 9.00), the male veterans (there are about 20 of us aged 37 to 70-ish) were sitting about having a cup of tea when one of our number, Brian Sweeney, told us he had been diagnosed with prostate cancer and was about to have a radical prostatectomy. We normally talk about football or cars or motorbikes or why Gordon Brown does that funny thing with his mouth or why we don't all square our blades over our thighs rather than our ankles. Anyway, we do not normally talk about prostate cancer. Men don't. Brian then told us that following a urinary infection in December 2004, he had a PSA test and the score was around 5; he had had another test in February, when it had risen to 7. Following a DRE and a biopsy, it was confirmed he had prostate cancer, and he was due to have an operation in mid-June. We all expressed our sympathy, or whatever you do in situations like that, and we all decided to have a PSA test. Of course, nobody did.

We don't mind getting up at 6.30 in the morning to drive across London to go rowing, but arranging to go and see a doctor is obviously beyond our abilities. The interesting thing is, with the benefit of hindsight, I'm sitting there unbeknown to me with a PSA reading probably already in triple figures, expressing my concern for Brian. Brian, hopefully, is one of the guys who got it early, gets it sorted and carries on with their lives, one of the reasons why there is now an 80 per cent cure rate if the disease is caught in what Professor Roger Kirby describes as the surgical 'window of curability'.

Anyway, roll the clock on to early August and now all we do is talk about prostate cancer. Well, that's not quite right, we do still bore on about why we don't all square our blades over our thighs rather than our ankles. It turns out five members of the club have or have had prostate cancer, as has the husband of the very nice lady who helps out behind the bar.

Doug got it at 47, diagnosed at a company medical, PSA 10, radical prostatectomy, doing very well, age now 54. Rob, 63, got it 4 years ago, company medical, PSA 32, radical prostatectomy, doing very well. Brian you know about, and the other guy prefers to keep stuff like this to himself. It's his way of dealing with the same stuff. He may be right.

Wednesday, 17 August 2005

I know I had said I wouldn't bother sending any more emails, but this is the one I sent out following my first visit to the Marsden at Sutton on 17 August 2005 – obviously my therapy route.

> Well, I've had so many anxious enquiries about the state of my motorbike following its accident on 8 July, even though I had promised to withdraw from further postings but being a self-obsessed attention seeker, here is a further update. However, this is self-evidently a wrong strategy. I know this because at a do last Saturday lunchtime, the lady sitting on my left-hand side, who I hadn't even been introduced to, let alone met before, well, she asked me how I was; and instead of giving her the short version of 'I could be dying but I'm very brave', I started giving her the long version. Would you believe it, instead of listening, if only out of politeness, about a tenth of the way into my epic of stoicism and bravery (mine) the fat cow said, 'Oh no, not another old man droning on about his illnesses.' We laughed.
>
> Still, the really good news is the Triumph Rocket 3 has come out of hospital and is back on the road. However, because I'm too lazy to chase after the very nice midwife that knocked Claudia and me off the bike on the A23, it still proudly carries some scars of battle. Claudia is back clubbing and the two ribs I cracked in my left back and the one in the front (revealed in an MRI spine scan) are now history, as is the embolism.
>
> So it's 17 August, the day of my first appointment at the Royal Marsden, Sutton. I'm anticipating some sort of epiphany, a definite St Paul on the road to Damascus (or was it Tarsus?) experience. Anyway, I'm driving up to Sutton in a biblical sort of way looking for some kind of medical route map. A state of grace.

Now, the really big problem with and in hospitals is nothing to do with MRSA bugs or waiting lists or patients or doctors or nurses. No, based on about two months of kicking around those sorts of institutions I can tell you the problem that affects everyone is in fact car parking. Tone, or rather Gordon, has lobbed money into the NHS, which means consultants now all drive top-of-the-range Mercedes. What's more, as every hospital is having what look like bolt-on toilet extensions and what with the building contractors' (two years old but big) BMWs, all the car-parking spaces are used up. So unless you want to pay £500 an hour for one of the five car-parking places remaining, you have to make alternative arrangements. I, by mistake (honest, guv), stumbled into the wrong but apparently free place.

So I'm sitting outside the urological oncology office. I'm shown into a small windowless cell with a sink, two chairs, a bed and a picture on the wall. A doctor walks in – young, obviously able, professional – and sees me; but actually I think he doesn't see me. He sees Mr 133-PSA-Test. I am defined by the number 133. I'd say that based on his experience and knowledge (considerable), he doesn't want to do stuff to me like surgery or even radiotherapy, because I'm Mr 133. He is maybe not wrong. Why suffer all the potential side effects if any potential benefit could be overtaken by events? Stay on the hormone treatment and in nine months or so, if the cancer hasn't spread to the spine or wherever else, then depending on the waiting list we may be able to offer radiotherapy. Have another PSA test before you go and I'll make another appointment in, say, two months' time.

So I'm sitting outside the urological oncology office waiting and the nurse fetches me again and I'm shown into the same small windowless cell with a sink, two chairs, a bed and a picture on the wall. A little, older, rounded man bounds in, Professor Dearnaley (I think). He just wants to say hello, he hasn't looked at my file or scans, some of which are still apparently en route from East Surrey Hospital, but he sees me, not Mr 133.

Tells me pretty much the same as the doctor about the potential short-term effects of hormone treatment and then says if it is appropriate they may be able to offer radiotherapy (IMRT) in January, which is about the right time, as after six months the hormone treatment should have shrunk the cancer cells to their minimum. He then says following the IMRT, for the next three years (no one has said years to me before) he'd like to keep me on hormone treatment to see the effects of hormone treatment post-radiotherapy. However, the long-term effects of hormone treatment can be diabetes, thinning bones, putting on weight, blah, blah – however, the best prevention is exercise. The little bouncy prof says, it would be useful for us to monitor you over this period, because you like exercise, although the tough bit is, however hard you exercise, the hormone treatment will reduce testosterone and your physical ability will be reduced. I like him.

He then gives me my fifth digital rectal examination (I don't like him that much) and says, about my prostate, that it isn't so impressive. I'm not too sure what he means. He then starts talking about a specific type of prostate cancer that is associated sometimes with high PSAs. I feel, cliché that it may be, that he hasn't got the answers but the next time I see him he may be asking the right questions. I have another PSA test and fix up to go back mid-September.

So, leaving the hospital, I'm thinking, who's right, done for by Christmas or I'll one day own a bus pass? And then I think, well, does it matter? I can hardly spend the next month asking the same question over and over again. The sun is shining, my ribs are better,

the embolism is gone, I've no symptoms, no side effects from the drugs, so get on with life and enjoy it and most important of all celebrate the fact you've used an NHS car park and there was no charge.
Andy
17 August 2005.

Well, that email covers the day. Before I leave, the Marsden very kindly arrange my next appointment. Arranging the patient's next appointment before he leaves is a simple but great idea. It makes you feel you belong and are in a continuing process. On my next visit to the Lingfield Surgery, on 31 August, I organise to do this with Lynne, too. She gives me another Zoladex injection, checks my INR and puts up my warfarin to 14 mg, before giving me the date of my next appointment with her. I'm to have the new PSA test on 5 September, so that I'll have the result in time for my next appointment at the Marsden: 3.30 p.m. on 14 September.

What is it, I reflect on my way home from the Marsden, about afternoon appointments in mid-September? At 3 p.m. on 15 September 1973, I had to face another rather nerve-racking appointment, but at least on that occasion I had 14 strapping Englishmen alongside me to help calm my fears as we ran out to face the All Blacks at Eden Park.

I didn't start playing rugby until I was 17 or 18 – I can't remember exactly. All I know is that from the moment I got the ball in my hands, the only thing I wanted to do was run and score tries. Mauling – of which there was a lot in the 1970s, not to mention fighting – didn't exactly turn me on, and scrums were an inconvenience that had to be tolerated. Stephen Jones, the long-serving and eminently readable rugby correspondent for the *Sunday*

Times, wrote a kind piece about me a while ago (was it a premature obituary, Jonesy?!) in which he said: 'Andy was a great player who played in the wrong era. England were absolutely abject at that time and with his ability, his athletic ability, if he had been launched properly he could have been perhaps the greatest lineout forward of all time.' Whenever you fancy a free lunch, Steve, give me a call.

But he's absolutely right. I would have loved to be playing the game today, certainly not for the money, because the professional game is primarily for the paying TV or real-time spectators and not for the players, which means you are an employee, a talented marionette, strings pulled by the coach. And yet, and yet . . . But anyway, it's a much faster and more fluid sport today and a hundred times more exciting to watch. In the 1970s, the game was so stop-start. What's the famous statistic from the 1963 match between Scotland and Wales? Something like 111 lineouts in 80 minutes – one every 43 seconds. Little wonder the BBC preferred to air *One Man and His Dog* and ITV chose Big Daddy and Giant Haystacks. Far more entertaining.

Anyway, as I said, I didn't start playing rugby until I was in my late teens, and I didn't take it seriously until the autumn of 1969, when I left the University of East Anglia and moved to London, where I joined Price Waterhouse as an articled clerk. I was renting a grotty little flat in Notting Hill (this was pre-Hugh Grant days, when not even dead people would be seen dead in the area) for ten quid a week.

I turned up at Rosslyn Park one day for a pre-season Saturday run-out for new members. At the time, they were one of the most prestigious clubs in the country, although they had no way of proving it. Hard as it might be to believe for anyone born after about 1980, up until 1987 there was no league rugby in England. So the clubs just sort of played each other in what were referred to somewhat ironically as friendly fixtures. We would play, say, the Wasps and all 12 sides from each club would play each other on the same Saturday, using the pitches at both clubs, usually with a dance in the evening. It was fun. There was also the knockout John Player Cup, which had started in 1972. The next step up from club competition was the County Championship, and it was from there that a player would usually be invited to the England trial game.

However, there was no lack of competitive edge to club rugby at the time, and there was certainly nothing amateur about the social side of things. In fact, in some ways, what increased your standing in your teammates' eyes wasn't your scrummaging or your sidestep but your ability to consume ten pints and a couple of ports and still remember the words to 'Inky Pinky Parlez-Vous'. But I loved that whole atmosphere, and I loved the Blazer Brigade, too, because you knew where you stood with them. They had a set of values and, sure, their values might not have been yours, but they stuck to them. They honestly believed they were preserving the soul of rugby union – which they did, until 26 August 1996 – and they were always kind to me. I always felt cherished.

After I joined Rosslyn Park I steadily worked my way up through the 4th XV, 3rd XV and 2nd XV until the big day arrived when I made my 1st XV debut. It was 6 December 1969, and I was playing number 8 against Richmond, for whom Chris Ralston – later to become a great friend and an England and Lions teammate – was playing in the second row. Tony Bucknall, the then England flanker, was in the back row.

Back then, global warming hadn't been invented and so, it being December, it was cold. Icy, too. In the first few minutes, displaying the sort of coordination for which I would later become famous, I slipped and landed on my kneecap. Ouch! Get up, Andy, give it a rub and continue. Don't want to blow your big chance. I limped round for the rest of the game, but after a shower, with the kneecap the size of a hot-air balloon, I took myself to hospital.

The X-ray confirmed that the kneecap had fractured in three places, but fortunately the doctor told me that because I was fit and young she wouldn't remove my kneecap. 'We'll let nature take its course.' My unrepayable debt to the medical profession began that day. The following summer, I was back training at full speed and raring to go for the 1970–71 season with Rosslyn Park. And it was during this season that I got my big break – and this time, luckily, it didn't involve bones.

I was invited to play for the Mickey Steele-Bodger's XV in one of their friendly fixtures against Cambridge University, the last big match for the university before the Varsity game. Mickey had been an England international in the late 1940s, and he had started this traditional fixture, which he still organises. Watching this particular game was John Reason, the patrician correspondent of the *Telegraph* at the time and a man roundly detested by the players, although that was only because he said it as it was and to hell with the consequences. John decided I would be good for England and began to sing my praises at every opportunity. Lucky me.

The following season, 1971–72, John more or less wrote me into the England trial, back then a quaint custom by which a team of Probables would play a team of Possibles, and then the selectors would gather round and pick names out of a hat. Or so the theory went.

I'd broken into the Middlesex team by now, so I was getting some good exposure in the County Championship, but it was still a shock to be selected at number 8 for our first match of the 1972 Five Nations. At Twickenham. Against Wales. J.P.R. Williams. Gerald Davies. Barry John. Gareth Edwards. Mervyn Davies. John Taylor. They were all legends, Grand Slam champions the previous year, and with a team that had formed the core of the 1971 Lions side that had beaten New Zealand. In the pack, Wales boasted 127 caps' worth of experience; England had 42, of which 21 belonged to hooker John Pullin.

At least my terror was eased slightly, ever so slightly, by the knowledge that five other players would be making their debuts alongside me: Mike Beese at centre, Alan Old and Jan 'Sprat' Webster at fly- and scrum-half respectively, Mike Burton at prop and Alan Brinn in the second row. Beese and Brinn didn't survive the season, but the rest of us managed to fool the selectors into inviting us back during the next few years.

Every rugby international will tell you that the first cap is special, and it's true. I'll never forget the moment when I emerged from the changing-room and sprinted onto the Twickenham pitch. It's addictive, I loved it . . . the noise, the smell, the adrenalin, everything . . . you just want it to last forever.

We knew we were massive underdogs, but Bob Hiller, our captain, exhorted us to tackle until we dropped, and that's exactly what we did. At first, our defence knocked the Welsh back, and we actually took the lead after half an hour when Bob kicked a penalty. Barry John then kicked two of his own before half-time, but as we sucked on our oranges, we began to think we might be able to beat Wales for the first time since 1963. 1963 . . . I was barely out of shorts then!

Unfortunately for us, as Wales sucked on their oranges, they must have been saying something along the lines of 'For Christ's sakes, lads, we haven't lost to these soft English bastards since 1963, so let's not do so today', because they scored a try not long after the restart.

They had a scrum on our 22 and Barry John drifted, nay glided, nay floated, towards the open side, getting himself into a position to drop a goal. That's what I expected, anyway. But suddenly JPR came steaming up the blind side, took a pass from Gareth Edwards and wham, bam, he was over for the try. And what, pray, was extra special about the try, and I don't mean that it condemned England to yet another defeat against Wales? It was the first international try worth four points to be scored at Twickenham. Ripley, you're part of rugby folklore, even if JPR did leave you trailing in his wake on his way to the try-line.

My second cap came against Ireland, who at the time were only marginally inferior to Wales. On this occasion, full-back Tom Kiernan was winning his 50th cap – the first Irish player to do so – and they also had the likes of Fergus Slattery, Willie John McBride, Ray McLoughlin, Ken Kennedy and Mike Gibson. We played above ourselves again and led from the moment Chris Ralston scored what would prove to be his one and only international try.

As the match moved into injury time, we were ahead 12–10, and an upset seemed probable until Kevin Flynn popped up on the wing to score and Kiernan added the conversion. My abiding memory of that match is that at some stage Tom Kiernan gave me his hand to pick me up off the ground – no words but a kind Irish smile. I loved him for that. However, that defeat demoralised us, and two weeks later we were annihilated 37–12 by France in Paris. We were embarrassing, conceding six tries and allowing France to rack up the most points ever scored by any team against England. The 25-point winning margin was also the biggest against an English side since Wales had beaten us 25–0 in 1905. As I sat in the dressing-room at the end of the match, I was so shattered I felt like I'd been born in 1905. It was the last game in the Stade Colombes, and the sun was on the French team.

We went to Edinburgh knowing that if we lost to a strong Scotland side, we would become the first England side to be whitewashed in the history of the Five Nations. Thoughts like that concentrate the mind, or they should do. They didn't for us. Several newspapers said afterwards that we ran out onto the pitch looking like a side that believed the match was already lost. They were right. Morale was at rock bottom, and when Peter Brown, Scotland's number 8, crashed over for a try, about five England players just stood and watched. The final score of 23–9 marked our heaviest defeat to Scotland in the Championship since 1901.

However, in spite of picking up the wooden spoon, there was a feeling, among the pack at least, that we had the makings of a pretty good unit. The selectorial chopping and changing during the season had happened mostly in the back line; up front we had remained largely intact. Mike Burton, Stack Stevens and John Pullin were a tough front row, with the immensely promising Fran Cotton challenging for a place, and Peter Dixon, Tony Neary and myself had enjoyed playing together in the back row and felt that we complemented each other well. Nonetheless, it was one thing to look forward to the 1973 Five Nations with optimism and another to have to board a plane to South Africa a few weeks after collecting the wooden spoon to play the Springboks at Ellis Park.

It was the first time England had toured South Africa, and whoever in the RFU (the English Rugby Football Union) had agreed to the itinerary had clearly never been on a rugby tour. Of any kind. Ever. Taking a squad of twenty-four players, we were to play seven matches in two and a half weeks, including games against three of South Africa's strongest provinces – Natal, Western Province and Northern Transvaal – ending with a Test match against the Springboks. If I'd had that wooden spoon to hand, I would have used it to hit the bloke who agreed to that schedule.

Nine of the squad were uncapped, among them a 28-year-old schoolteacher from Moseley called Sam Doble. Sam was a big lad with a mop of blond hair who'd started out as a number 8 before converting to full-back. He didn't take himself, or life, too seriously, which perhaps goes some way to explaining why he hadn't played for England earlier.

The tour opener was against Natal in Durban, a city I fell in love with straight away. Great weather, great beaches and great surf. Just keep an eye out for the great whites. I also found that the hard dry pitches of South Africa suited my game much more than the soggy muddy swamps that were common in Europe at the time. I could run to my heart's content. To totally blow my own trumpet, I was superb against Natal, but then so was the entire pack. We creamed Natal 19–0 and scored three tries along the way. Three tries! We'd only scored two during the previous Five Nations Championship.

Three days later, we played Western Province in Cape Town. Now, I'd been led to believe that Durban and Cape Town were the two most Anglophile cities in South Africa. And there was me thinking Welsh supporters had cornered the market in insults. But it had little effect on us as we made it two wins out of two. Two days later (yes, two days later), we won our third tour match, and two days after that we won our fourth. So let's do some sums here. We played the tour opener against Natal on 17 May and seven days later we played and won our fourth match. And modern players moan about burnout.

We had three days' rest before our fifth provincial game, the toughest yet, against Northern Transvaal. Their pack was the strongest in South Africa, and guys like Williams in the second row and Van Wyk the hooker were experienced Springboks. We were also now on the high veldt, where the air is thinner and the people blonder, although the reason we were trailing 13–3 midway through the second half was probably because of the former. John Pullin gathered the pack round him and ordered us in his strong West Country accent to pull our bloody fingers out in the last quarter. It was also the moment that Chris Ralston told me I was too soft and too nice for Test rugby. He was right, of course, but to spite Chris I decided to act 'hard' for what was left of the game.

Sam Doble, who'd been in outstanding form the whole tour, kicked two long-range penalty goals, and then, with just a few minutes remaining, I got the ball in the Northern Transvaal 22 and thundered towards the try-line. Was I reciting Tennyson's 'Charge of the Light Brigade' as I ran? I can't remember. Probably. Unfortunately, Sam couldn't convert the try and so the match finished a 13-all draw. We won our final warm-up match three days later, and then had the luxury of four days – four whole days! – before the Test match.

There were four new caps in the England side, including Sam Doble at full-back and John Watkins on the flank, and we were facing a South African team who were unbeaten in their last seven matches. Not only had they beaten the All Blacks twice, but they'd tonked France 22–9 in Bloemfontein the previous season. As the French had humiliated us a few weeks earlier in the Five Nations, we were given as much chance of success as a Frenchman keeping a vow of celibacy.

But within the England squad there was an air of quiet

confidence. The tour had really bonded us, and we enjoyed each other's company; crucially, of course, there was no pressure on us. It wasn't if we were going to lose, according to the press, it was by how many points. But we ran out onto the pitch believing we would win. And we did. We didn't just win, we stuffed the Springboks. Jan Webster and Alan Old were magnificent at half-back, cool and calm and always taking the right decision, and me, Watkins and Neary at full-back were all over the place. Don't believe it? Well, two of the Springbok back row that day were never picked again, such was our dominance!

The hero, however, was big Sam Doble. He kicked four penalties in our 18–9 win, including a couple from inside his own half. That was practically unheard of in those days, because balls were much heavier than today, but Sam had some boot on him. He also converted the only try of the match, a real beauty by Alan Morley, our winger, in the corner. Sam's 14 points were the most scored by an individual player in a match between England and South Africa and equalled the English record for any match, set by Bob Hiller against France in 1971.

Tragically, that was the peak of Sam's rugby career. He won two more caps the following season, but then, I think, he declined to travel to Dublin to play Ireland because of terrorist threats, and he was out on his ear. Four years later, he died of cancer aged thirty-three. But I haven't forgotten your big boot, Sam, and nor have quite a few South Africans!

The 1973 Five Nations will be remembered as the year when Dublin gave 15 Englishmen a standing ovation and then proceeded to trample all over us! The previous season, Wales and Scotland had refused to travel to Ireland for their fixtures because of threats of violence from terrorist organisations. By doing so they probably denied Ireland the opportunity to win the Grand Slam, because they had beaten us and the French away and would have been hard to beat on home soil.

Although the England team received similar threats in 1973, we had no intention of pulling out, despite starting the Five Nations with a thumping from Wales in Cardiff. It wasn't that we'd played badly; the Welsh were just too good for us, and the last of their five tries, scored by John Bevan, was a gem. Ten of the side handled the ball before Bevan put us out of our misery. It was one of those tries you just sit back and admire, even if you're on the opposing side!

So, three weeks later, we went to Dublin, and in true English fashion we concealed our apprehension beneath humour. We played musical chairs whenever we travelled on the team bus, reasoning that the dozens of IRA snipers perched on the rooftops would find it harder to hit one of us if we were always swapping seats.

When we ran out onto Lansdowne Road, the Irish supporters cheered us to the rafters. Of all the British teams, England had perhaps most reason to fear terrorist attack, and yet here we were, fulfilling our fixture. The Irish were grateful – for as long as it took for the referee to start the match. Then they let us have it. Willie John McBride was winning his 50th cap that day, and he was madder than usual. But we stuck to it, even though Ireland were clearly the better side, and the 18–9 scoreline was a fair reflection on the difference between the teams. It was England's seventh successive Five Nations defeat, and as John Pullin said in the shortest and the most memorable post-match dinner speech I have ever heard, 'We may not be very good, but at least we turn up.'

But then we won our next game, beating France 14–6, and the one after that, in which we defeated Scotland

20–13. Two wins on the trot . . . oh, the giddy heights of success! It actually meant that we finished top of the Five Nations, along with Wales, Ireland, France and Scotland. All five teams had won two from two – the first time it had happened. We might have had the worst points difference, but who cared?! England had finished top. Sort of.

That summer we were scheduled to tour Argentina, but the trip was cancelled at the last minute because of terrorist threats. Who exactly the terrorists were, I was never sure, and what a group of English rugby players – and not very good ones at that – had done to incur their wrath I was even less clear on. But the RFU decided it was too dangerous and cancelled the tour. Great, we all thought, a summer off. Let's go to the beach. Whoah, not so fast, said the RFU, we'll find somewhere to tour. OK, we thought, what about Hawaii or Mauritius or the Seychelles? Where did we go? New Zealand. Gee, thanks.

We left England in late August, stopped off at Fiji just as flash floods hit the island, so we were unable to train because the practice ground was covered with hundreds of frogs, washed up out of the creeks and crevices by the heavy rain. Three days after arriving in Fiji, we played an unofficial Test against their national XV and thrashed them, er, 13–12. It was better than it sounds, in fact, seeing as our bodies were telling us that it wasn't mid-afternoon, it was in fact the middle of the night and we should be sleeping, not playing rugby in extreme humidity.

From Fiji we flew to New Zealand, exchanging the sauna of Suva for the winter chill of New Plymouth. Not surprisingly, we lost 6–3 to Taranaki in our first provincial match, and four days later we were whipped 25–16 by Wellington. Three days after that, it was Canterbury's turn, and their 19–12 win meant we went into the one-off Test against the All Blacks at Eden Park without a win in

New Zealand. We started to wish we were in Argentina, terrorists and all.

England and New Zealand had played each other nine times before our match, and England had only one miserly victory to our name, a 13–0 victory in 1936 – and that had been at Twickenham. Who gave us any chance of making it two from ten? Well, the 15 blokes wearing white shirts on 15 September 1973. Even though we had lost all our provincial matches, we knew that our Test team, particularly our forward pack, could match the All Blacks. Colin Meads had retired a season or two before, and probably only their flanker and captain, Ian Kirkpatrick, could have been called world class, whereas we had at least three players who fitted that bill in our scrum: John Pullin, Fran Cotton and Tony Neary. We also had a rapidly improving Roger Uttley in the second row and yours truly at number 8. But the man of the match was John Watkins, the Gloucester blind-side, winning his fourth cap. He was magnificent: everything you expect from a hard, tough, hairy Gloucester forward, with the kindest of hearts.

Behind the pack, Jan Webster had his best-ever game for England, completely eclipsing the far more experienced Sid Going and providing the catalyst for all three of our tries. 'Sprat', we called Jan, because he was more or less that size; but his heart was out of all proportion to the rest of him.

The All Blacks were outmanoeuvred at every turn, and they were lucky to get away with a 16–10 defeat. We had a couple of tries disallowed and deserved a bigger winning margin. But, hey, who's complaining? We had become the first English side – the first home nation – to win a Test in New Zealand. No other national side was to achieve this in the twentieth century, which says something about the power of All Black rugby over time.

The RFU, in their wisdom, had arranged to have us on a flight home the evening of our victory – they had probably envisaged a sound thumping and deemed it prudent to have us on the first flight out of Auckland. As we drove to the airport, our tour manager, Sandy Saunders, asked us to quieten down for a moment because he had something to say. 'Boys,' he said, 'you have stolen the crown jewels of rugby. Remember this day, because you will dine out on it forever.' And do you know, he was right. Although I played for England for another two years, nothing that followed compared to those two victories in South Africa and New Zealand. I've been dining out on them ever since, particularly that win against the mighty All Blacks. 15 September 1973. What a day.

14 September 2005. What sort of day will that be? The day of my next appointment at the Marsden, the outcome of which would depend largely on my next PSA result. So before we get there, perhaps I should tell you what I think about that measurement which has taken on so much importance in the past few weeks.

My Take on the PSA Test

As far as I can see, the PSA test has two functions: the first is as part of the less than perfect toolkit for diagnosing prostate cancer; the second is as a monitoring tool to identify the progression or regression of the disease in the patient. In this case, me. As a single, stand-alone number it obviously has some value, but that value becomes much greater when it is part of a series of numbers. When the PSA test is being used to identify the rate of change, clearly more importance can be attached to it.

The PSA is a blood test. The acronym stands for prostate

specific antigen, which is an enzyme, the supercharger that turns the jelly with fluid secreted by the two seminal vesicles into liquid semen before ejaculation. The sperm itself is produced by the testicles, which also make the male hormone testosterone. The PSA can enter the bloodstream, sometimes because cancerous cells are weakening the walls of the prostate, enabling PSA to escape into the bloodstream. If this is the case, the cancerous cells themselves may also seep out and seed themselves in the soft tissue around the prostate, the most likely landing places being nearby or distant lymph nodes and the base of the spine. The higher the seepage, the bigger the PSA count. But does a high count indicate the presence of cancer? Not necessarily. But it is a warning sign and does mean that further tests should be done.

According to an article published in the *Observer Magazine* on 8 May 2005, 'Gland on the Run' by Simon Garfield:

> In the US, about 70 per cent of men over 50 know their PSA scores, compared with 3 per cent in the UK. In this country the incidence of prostate cancer is higher than any other (in 2001, 30,140 men were diagnosed, accounting for 22 per cent of all new cancer reports in men), but death rates are still some way behind those of lung cancer, due to the relatively successful rates of intervention if detected early . . . The official line from the Department of Health, supported to some degree by Cancer Research UK, is that we don't yet have clear evidence that PSA testing saves lives.

Garfield's article was a piece about Tony Elliot, 58, *Time Out* publisher, who in mid-January 2005 went to see his doctor following a dizzy spell and a temporary loss of memory. He was given a thorough going over, including a PSA test, the result of which was 5.4. It doesn't say, but I presume he was given a DRE. A short while later, he underwent a biopsy. The article doesn't give Tony's Gleason score (hardly surprising, this is space filler for a Sunday mag, not a medical report). Tony had a radical prostatectomy, carried out by Professor Robert Kirby, on 8 March at The London Clinic. According to the article, his prostate was 40 cc (normal would be 20 cc) of which 7.6 cc was cancer. At the time the article was written, in April, he had recovered about 80 per cent of bladder control and the surgeon had told him, if necessary, he will supply him with Viagra in a few months.

So clearly the PSA test can be extremely valuable; however, it can be unreliable as an indicator of cancer. BPH (benign prostatic hyperplasia, the medical term for enlargement of the prostate in older men) and prostatitis, the inflammation of the prostate, neither of which are carcinogenic, may also lead to an increased PSA, although there is no associated spread of cancer cells as there are no cancer cells to spread. However, prostate cancer usually causes a more dramatic rise in PSA levels. It's the rate of change rather than the single number which is the most credible measurement.

On the other hand, read almost any article or textbook, and the same point is repeatedly made, although the percentages may vary: that 'one in four prostate cancers do not cause an elevation in PSA'. (*The ABCs of Prostate Cancer* by J.E. Oesterling & M.A. Moyad, referred to hereafter as *ABC*). Garfield's article records that during a speech to the National Prostate Cancer Conference in 2004, Professor Kirby, one of the country's foremost experts on the disease:

> mentioned that some people have taken to referring to PSA as 'promotion of stress and anxiety'. He also said that, unfortunately, the PSA test is not even a good indicator of

negative results. Research published last year suggests that of those people in the study who had a PSA of less than 4, 17 per cent did already have prostate cancer.

One fact is clear, however: PSA tends to rise with age. There is a widespread use of age-specific reference ranges, and it's also taken into account that normal PSA values differ slightly between the races. What is normal? Well, if the traditional normal PSA range is between 0 and 4 ng/ml, the upper limit of normal could be as low as 2 for an Asian 40–49-year-old man but as high as 6.5 for a black or white 70–79-year-old man.

However, for me, at 133 there is little comfort: 'regardless of age and race, however, PSA levels greater than 10 ng/ml are a pretty accurate sign of prostate cancer, research shows that 70–80% of those who have a test result this high are found to have the disease' (*ABC*).

Also, the two lines on page 16 of Prof Kirby's book, *Small Gland, Big Problem*, hit pretty hard: 'if cancer is to be identified at a stage when it is still curable, then it should be detected before the PSA rises much above 10 ng/ml.' Cripes! At 133, I'm not only outside the window of curability, quite frankly, it seems I'm not even in the building. Probably not even in the same postal district as the building, according to a throwaway quote from Prof Kirby's anaesthetist Dr Amoroso in the *Observer* article. He is railing against the fact that in one fairly recent year the amount of government money put towards prostate-cancer research was just £47,000.

That's crap, that's enough for a tiny project. Now it's about £4 million, which is still a drop in the ocean. Every hospital in the UK is littered with men with prostate cancer and secondary deposits, who are put on hormones, which gives them big boobs, no sex life, and they are going to die in two years.

Lawks, that's me! And with an initial PSA count of 133, perhaps even two years is being hugely optimistic. I suppose I'll find out in due course.

So to sum up (although I intend coming back to the PSA test), the PSA is useful in helping to diagnose prostate cancer, particularly over time, as the rate of change tells us more than a one-off test. When it's done in conjunction with a DRE and a biopsy, it is likely that if you have prostate cancer, it will be found, and if the detection is early enough and you are young enough to make it worthwhile, surgery will be a viable option.

It is possible, of course, that you could have a PSA test that is not abnormally high for your age and race, an inconclusive DRE test and a biopsy that fails to hit the cancerous cells and be told you do not have prostate cancer when you do. Which would be a bit of a bugger. However, it is quite likely, as you are in the game, that you will have another PSA test, and this one may show a disproportionate increase, and, again, if the detection is early enough and you are young enough to make it worthwhile, surgery would still be a viable option.

So PSA tests are particularly useful not so much in the detection of the disease, although they obviously have their place, but in the post-surgery, radiotherapy, check-up phase. Each sequential test will be a strong marker as to whether the disease has permanently or merely temporarily regressed or progressed, and it is the rate of change that is the crucial factor.

There is also, I imagine, a time when the PSA test is not particularly relevant as it is only too obvious to the patient that the disease has spread.

Monday, 5 September 2005

We're pretty much up to date now, and I'm writing in real time. I've just had my weekly INR test and am now on 14 mg of warfarin. Today, at the Lingfield Surgery, I had my blood taken for the PSA test, the result of which Prof Dearnley had asked me to take to the Marsden on Wednesday, 14 September at 3.30 p.m. I can pick up the new PSA score on Thursday, 8 September.

My first blood test was around 18 June, and I was given the result on 20 June at 133. My second was on 14 July and the result was 95. This, apparently, was OK and moving in the right direction. The biopsy would probably have irritated the prostate, raising the count, so the score may not have accurately reflected the effects of the hormone treatment. My third blood test was at the Marsden on 17 August. They must have the result, but I am too frightened to want to know. My fourth blood test was today and I can pick up the result on 8 September.

Well, I'm scared. Why am I scared? If the PSA is not responding to the hormone treatment, then presumably the option of radiotherapy is likely to be less relevant in my case than I and Prof Dearnley had hoped. Now, at any stage you could worry about anything, and goodness knows there is enough to worry about. Picking up, as I am, dog ends of information from the Net and probably reading things out of context could lead, if you let it, to a really miserable time.

For instance, in the *ABC* book on page 83 under 'Fast Fact' we have: 'The majority (95%) of prostate cancers are called adenocarcinomas. Less than 5% are non-adenocarcinomas, which are usually much more aggressive and do not respond to any type of hormone treatment.' Cripes, maybe I've got that! Stick that on top of the

10 ng/ml window of curability and the two years of getting fat, being impotent and dying – and, well, you could get yourself into a bit of a state. There is no point and one can only come back to the view, don't bother worrying, because why waste the precious time between now and whenever and whatever?

It was also obvious to me when I was shown the MRI scan on 14 July that, although the oncologist was evidently good at his trade, he could not say with absolute certainty if the indications of possible localised cancer were in fact merely that – possible indications. And if he could not say that, neither could he say with certainty how fast the cancer would grow or if it would become more aggressive with time.

It is also quite possible that a cancer could go from a curable state to an incurable state even without any noticeable change in the PSA, and it is unlikely that you would be scanned so often as to pick up each and every change. You wanna worry, then there is fertile ground for sinking into some abyss or other. I can only repeat myself, more for me than you: don't bother worrying, because why waste the precious time between now and whenever and whatever.

However, hope is a good thing, and why will I go and pick up my PSA test this Thursday? Because I might as well know and then just deal with it. Ian Dury had that little number, 'Reasons to be Cheerful', before he popped his clogs and Bob Marley sang 'Don't worry 'bout a thing, 'cause every little thing is gonna be all right' before some nasty disease swept him away. They probably knew what was happening to them and dealt with it.

Wednesday, 7 September 2005

I don't know, but I feel this week will shed more light on the questions:

1.   Is the cancer still confined to the prostate?
2.   Has it migrated to other reproductive organs near the prostate?
3.   Has it spread to the lymph nodes, nearby?
4.   Has it spread to the lymph nodes, distant?
5.   Has it travelled to the bones?

In one week's time, I will go to the Marsden for the second time. The first occasion, in August, was really just to say hello, but by now they should have got all the scans sent to them, looked at them, hopefully read the various reports and reached their own judgement. I am probably a five-minute discussion amongst their many discussions, but I feel they will do the best for me, which could be, in response to the five questions above, stay on the hormones and see what happens or they could confirm a date, perhaps in January, to start the IMRT or maybe even some other course of action.

In the meantime, tomorrow I pick up the PSA test.

In spite of non-adenocarcinomas and the 10 ng/ml window of curability and the two years of getting fat, being impotent and dying, I am feeling sort of confident. Why's that, Andrew?

Well, first off, there's Dr Charlotte Foley's article, 'Chemotherapy for Hormone-Escaped Prostate Cancer – A New Gold Standard', for the Prostate Research Campaign UK newsletter. She starts the article with the sentence: 'Once prostate cancer has spread to the bones, it is incurable.' Now, according to my bone scan of 20 June, my cancer has not spread to the bones, so maybe it's curable.

Second, I've had five DRE tests to date, and neither the ward doctors, the urologist nor the oncologist at East Surrey or Prof Dearnley seemed to be particularly impressed by my prostate as being dramatically abnormal.

Third, the **Gleason score**. Because apparently not all prostate cancers look or act the same, after a biopsy the pathologist examines tissue specimens from the two most representative areas of the tumour and assigns a grade between 1 (cancer is not very aggressive and is unlikely to spread quickly) and 5 (likely to grow fast). The two grades that occur most often in the sample are then recorded and added together to give an overall score of 2 to 10.

It is possible, however, that a tumour with a high Gleason score (8–10) will not increase a man's PSA level dramatically, because these cancers act very differently from normal prostate tissue and do not release as much PSA. On the other hand, some tumours with low Gleason scores (2–4) can dramatically increase a man's PSA level, as these cancers look and act similar to normal prostate tissue and release PSA. The pathologist's report gave my Gleason score as 7 (4 + 3). Moderate-grade cancers, presumably, can produce significant quantities of PSA, while others might not change the PSA level at all. Of course, although it's objective as far as I and the doctors are concerned, the actual score reflects the subjective view of the pathologist. They could get it wrong.

Whereas the Gleason score seems to be a universal marker, there are also various other staging systems which deal with how aggressive the cancer is and how far it has spread. The one most referred to seems to be TNM (T for Tumour, N for Nodes, M for Metastasis). I am not too sure about my own relative scores, but I'll ask Prof Dearnley about them next week.

Fourth, I am feeling good. I don't seem to have any symptoms and am experiencing no side effects from the hormone treatment. Actually, that's not right. I have stopped waking up with an erection and have little interest in sex. I have started, for the first time in my life, to put on weight around the stomach, but if I stop eating so much and do a bit more exercise, maybe that's the answer. The usual dieting advice: move around more, eat less.

Fifth and finally, for some reason, I have taken great comfort in a conversation I had with Dr Sneddon, the cardio surgeon on Holmwood Ward who took care of me when I had the pulmonary embolism. After he had passed me on to the urologists, but before I left East Surrey Hospital on 25 June, I met him by chance in the ward corridor. He asked me how I was, I said fine. He then said, 'You do realise that taking these hormone tablets, when this is all over, will probably impact your 2,000-m indoor-rowing times.'

There I was, worrying about not being around in two years, but his concern was that as a result of all this stuff my 2,000-m indoor-rowing times might suffer. For some reason I found his concern about this possible side effect massively comforting.

Thursday, 8 September 2005

Today, another 100 men in the UK will be told they have prostate cancer. The first day of the final and fifth Ashes test match at the Oval, where my two girls are taking pictures of the punters for Red Snappers (a marketing company who specialise in photographing live events like big sporting occasions) to earn some money for a week's holiday before they go back to university. The day I am due to pick up my 5 September PSA test.

It's rather like awaiting the results of some school examination. I don't know much about prostate cancer, but I'm learning fast. Lynne at the Lingfield Surgery told me as she injected the Zoladex into my stomach on 4 August, 'This'll sort you out.' I'm still not too sure what she meant.

However, I would like to consider a hypothetical question. I now know cancers take different forms, grow at different rates and have different characteristics. For a moment however let's imagine that the rate of growth is uniform and that this is reflected in the PSA which, say, doubles every year. So working backwards: in June 2005 my PSA was 133; in June 2004 it would have been 64; in June 2003, 32; in June 2002, 16; and so on, down to 8 then 4 then 2 then 1 then 0.5 ng/ml. Which takes me to June 1997. Now, I know this is a highly unlikely sequence, but it lets me, within this arbitrary structure, pose three very basic questions.

1.   Would I have wanted to know my PSA earlier than 24 June 2005?
2.   Why did I get prostate cancer?
3.   What caused it?

Well, in reverse order, like the contestants for a medically incorrect beauty pageant, here goes.

What caused it?
Well, I haven't got the answer to that and neither as yet has mankind, although medicine has made huge strides in treatment, particularly if cancers are found early, and in palliative care and pain relief.

Cancers or tumours are the result of a breakdown in genetic control. Cells divide as and when the body needs them to; however, if cells begin dividing (who knows why?) in an unregulated manner, then the mass of unregulated cells form a tumour. If this tumour has the ability to invade surrounding healthy tissue, it is cancerous. Cells can break off from the original invasive tumour and enter the bloodstream or lymphatic system, developing secondary cancers in other parts of the body.

When medical research finds out about the breakdown in genetic control, it will also discover what caused my and every other cancer.

Why did I get prostate cancer?
Well, obviously there was a breakdown in my genetic control and cells in my prostate began dividing in an unregulated manner. But why me, Lord?

I've read the books (well, some of them) and the articles (one or two), and I've come to the conclusion it shouldn't have happened to me and it's all a bit of a mistake. However, first of all, a few general points.

First, this is (essentially but not always) an old man's disease, but as life expectancy in the OECD (Organisation for Economic Co-operation and Development) countries has moved from about 50 to 80 during the last 100 years and methods of detection have improved, the numbers of men identified to be suffering from prostate cancer have risen. It is likely to become the most common malignancy in men.

One of my sisters, Jackie, married Frank Andoh, a Ghanaian, in the 1960s. I have a nephew, aged 40, now living in LA. As I, his uncle, have prostate cancer, Yeofi, being black and aged 40, should be thinking about taking a PSA test and having a DRE now. In fact, I'll phone him up and tell him, which will really cheer him up. There are two reasons why Yeofi should do this, detailed below as points two and three.

Second, race and ethnicity. The article 'Cancer statistics, 1996' (*A Cancer Journal for Clinicians*) showed that the percentage of deaths due to prostate cancer in the US according to race and ethnicity were: Asians and Pacific Islanders, 4 per cent; Hispanics, Native Americans and whites, 6 per cent; and African Americans 9 per cent. Proportionately, black men seem to get hit earlier (40+) than white and Asian men (50+).

Third, according to *ABC* (p. 10), the greater the number of family members who have had the disease, the higher the risk not only of getting the disease but of developing it earlier. The average man's risk of getting prostate cancer is between 10 and 15 per cent (I don't know where they get this figure from). If another single family member has had prostate cancer, the risk is double. If two family members have had prostate cancer, the risk becomes two to five times higher. The bad news for my nephew Yeofi is that his uncle, me, has prostate cancer; the good news is that the other male members of my family on my father's and mother's side all lived into their 80s, and my elder brother, 65, has had the PSA test and is 0.5 ng/ml.

Fourth, there is a theory that exposure to ultraviolet radiation from the sun has a protective effect against prostate cancer. I love the sun.

Fifth, a diet high in saturated fats apparently increases the risk of prostate cancer, whereas a diet containing plenty of fibre has the opposite effect. Tomatoes (which are a source of the antioxidant lycopene), especially the skins, and fish (which contains vitamin D) seem to have their adherents.

Finally, listed in all the books, there are all the usual

suspects, which all of us already know about by the time we're of an age to worry about prostate cancer. Obesity doesn't help and neither does smoking, neither does drinking more than 22 units of alcohol per week.

In fact, if, once you've been diagnosed, you can't smoke, drink or eat what you like and you're probably sexually dysfunctional, you've got to at least ask the third question.

Would I have wanted to know earlier than 24 June 2005?
Well, of course, it depends.

If the result of the PSA test I pick up today is, say, below 20, I will probably be given the radiotherapy treatment at the Marsden and maybe, just maybe, I get cured. However, there are potential side effects associated with radiotherapy, effects such as impotence, incontinence and the concern that the cancer hasn't been fully cleaned out and may be looking for a return match – a state of anxiety that would also have existed if I had found out prior to 24 June 2005. To that date I had no anxiety or symptoms. In fact, the last seven years have been brilliant.

If the result of the PSA test today is bad, and next week the indications are I've missed the last train to Cure City, then I'll just have to deal with it and hypothetical questions will become invalid, because I will have no choice. On balance, however, if it is possible I may be cured, then I'm glad I didn't find out I had prostate cancer until I did. I'd prefer to be treated at a point when a cure is still possible (maybe now) but to have deferred the side effects as long as possible, including that of anxiety. Still following this?

I'll get a clue today.

Later, 8 September 2005

Actually, I won't. I've just been to Lingfield Surgery, and the very nice receptionist told me, 'Sorry, dear, nothing has come in yet, try again on Monday, 12 September.' Here I am, chewing my fingernails. Oh well, you gotta roll with the punches.

This also allows me to continue with my medically improbable hypothetical theory of the PSA doubling every year. Let's look forward from 20 June, when the result of my first PSA, at 133, was given to me. I had no symptoms or pain from the cancer. If I had not had a pulmonary embolism, I certainly wouldn't have gone to the doctor just, for instance, out of curiosity. My approach to medicine has always been, 'Don't bother anyone, just get on with life, it'll get better.'

So, looking forward, what might have happened to me? Well, in June 2006, my PSA would have been, according to my totally hypothetical theory of annual doubling, 266, and the following year 532. However, by this time, if not before, I would probably have been in such pain, likely chronic back pain, that even I would have gone to the doctor, and although the medical profession could have done something – they are brilliant, they can always do something – it would have been beyond their considerable ability to do much other than reduce the pain.

As it is, right now I'm still in this uncertain area, where maybe a cure is still just possible. I suppose, in this ambiguous place which I am now in, the most common symptom of prostate cancer is no symptom at all.

I'm starting to think about the 7.55 theory. Which is this: for years, each weekday I caught the 7.55 from Lingfield station to London Bridge. My idea of success was to be dropped off at the station at about 7.54 and 45 seconds and walk onto the platform just as the train was pulling into the station. No time wasted. I could, instead of hanging about on the platform, be at home eating toast and listening to the radio and annoying Elisabeth and the kidlets. My time. I didn't want to get to the station at, say, 7.50 and just wait. Neither, of course, did I want to get to the station just as the train was pulling out. I usually made it. I much preferred to have my time and risk missing the 7.55. Sometimes, of course, the 7.55 was late – that was OK – or never arrived at all. I can't ever remember it being early.

Now, here's the complication: I feel obliged to tell those at risk to take a PSA test and have a DRE test. However, there may be no need to arrive at the station at 7.50 and kick your heels and be anxious. Myself, I feel, possibly wrongly, that if I get away with 133, whatever that means, then I have arrived at the station at 7.54 and 45 seconds and have not during my 50s, which have been great, been anxious or troubled. It's heretical (and possibly ironic, if I have missed the 7.55), but maybe I wouldn't have wanted to know before now, because I have had my time, it hasn't been stolen by prostate cancer.

Monday, 12 September 2005

Midday, and England are 100 for 3 in the final day of the Fifth Test at the Oval. Kevin Pietersen facing Shane Warne. At stake, the Ashes – the same Ashes that England last held in 1989. Result uncertain. It must be catching.

Anyway, I've just got back from Lingfield Surgery, where Lynne did an INR test (2.1 and still 14 mg of warfarin). Before that, I asked the receptionist if she had my PSA result back as I needed to take a print-out to the Marsden on Wednesday, 14 September. She checked on her computer and said yes, it was 1.1 and she would do me a print-out. I told her I didn't want the INR score but the PSA result. She

looked at me and said we don't have the most recent INR
reading, but this is your PSA result from the blood test on
5 September.

I sat down and said thank you.

How could it be 1.1? I had hoped it would be lower than
the last time, although admittedly I'd been too scared to
find out what the result was last time.

First test, 20 June, 133; second, 14 July, 95; third, 17
August, too scared to ask. Today, 1.1. I didn't know what
this meant. The DREs had always been, in the words of
Prof Dearnley, 'That isn't so impressive.' But the biopsy
had shown a Gleason score of 7, and, in the words of
Mr Swinn, based on the pathologist's verbal report, 'It's
unequivocal. You have prostate cancer.'

I phoned up the Marsden to find out the 17 August result,
just to see if there had been a mistake, if I had someone
else's result and, scarily for them, they had mine. I was
put through to the urology department, and I asked if it
was possible to have my PSA result from the 17 August
test. They are not allowed to give out PSA results over
the phone, which I can fully understand. I explained my
situation, and the voice at the end of the phone said she
could tell me it was nearer my most recent test. So 1.1
wasn't a mistake. But what, if anything, did it mean? I keep
looking at the print-out. I think it is good, but though I
don't want to cross Anxiety Bridge, neither do I want to
give myself false hope. No, the answer is the same as when
I left the Marsden hospital on 17 August:

> So, leaving the hospital, I'm thinking, who's right,
> done for by Christmas or I'll one day own a bus pass?
> And then I think, well, does it matter? I can hardly
> spend the next month asking the same question
> over and over again. The sun is shining, my ribs
> are better, the embolism is gone, I've no symptoms,

no side effects from the drugs, so get on with life and enjoy it and most important of all celebrate the fact you've used an NHS car park and there was no charge.

Don't do troughs and crests. Enjoy today. Expect nothing beyond what is. Be yourself. As Voltaire suggested through Candide, cultivate your own garden. False hope is as dangerous as anxiety. I can almost feel an attack of Rudyard Kiplingism coming on.

Platitudes and clichés rule OK. But when you're considering your own mortality, they seem strangely apposite as does the 'If you've got good health and a few friends then maybe you're ahead of the game and you don't need much more' school of thought.

I'll put the print-out aside and wait for Prof Dearnley to tell me what is what on Wednesday, and in the meantime maybe go watch the cricket.

Tuesday, 13 September 2005

Actually, without straying into hierarchy-of-needs territory (physical, emotional and spiritual), you do need something other than good health and a few friends, and that is money.

Now, you can come at this from a variety of standpoints. The most recent approach for me was what I did the first week I was out of hospital in late June. Then, everything seemed urgent. What would have happened if I had died of the pulmonary embolism? And when I asked Mr Swinn on 24 June, 'How long have I got?', he could have said anything. So the first thing I did was to tackle all those financial things I ought to have dealt with but had left undone, obviously for the very good reason that there was always something better to do. There's always something better to be done than to organise the few pathetic assets that you have gathered around you.

So when I left hospital, I put together a folder listing details of assets, obligations and then drew up a will and asked a friend to act as executor. In this same mood, I then emptied all those boxes which you collect over 57 years and had a wonderful few days wandering down Amnesia Avenue and clearing things up. After that, I found myself going through all my clothes and taking some of them to the Oxfam shop. Actually, it was at this juncture that I decided to stop. You can take this impending death stuff too far.

The next angle on money is, what are your financial circumstances? I cannot imagine what it is like to be a single mum on benefits on a sink estate with some nasty malignant disease or other. Let alone financially, how do you even begin to cope?

My children are now almost able to support themselves financially. Prostate cancer is an older man's disease and the financial demands of middle-aged people are reduced. I'm self-employed and I get by. But for some, a major issue in dealing with cancer must be dealing with the changed and changing financial outlook.

Wednesday, 14 September 2005

I go to the Marsden, clutching my PSA test, full of expectation. After my visit, I send out another email.

> The Prostate Kid was anxious. Anxious but cool. He was wearing his black jeans, black polo shirt and leather jacket. The Kid dismounted and left his slightly bruised 2,300-cc motorcycle at the Royal Marsden hitching post. The Kid noticed the park was full, but bein' on his cycle, he wasn't payin'. Yeah, the Kid was

cool all right. The Kid was also now impotent. Three months of hormone treatment had smashed his PSA from 133 to 1.1 and given him, apparently, an extended life and a limp dick. The Kid was kinda grateful.

The Kid strode (the Kid never just walked) to the reception desk and took his turn. The Kid was kinda hopin' to see the Prof, but the Doc walked in.

On 17 August, the Doc hadn't seen the Kid, he'd just seen Mr 133. Now, on 14 September, again the Doc didn't see the Kid, or even Mr 133; he now saw Mr T3aN1M0. Which means, in doc-speak, tumour grade 3a (on a scale of 1–4), spread to local lymph nodes (N1, on a scale of 0–3) but not to distant sites (M0). The Doc had obviously been at work checking through the scans. The Doc was good, very good, but the Kid couldn't help but feel like just another of the 100 men who are told each day in the UK they have prostate cancer, and the Kid wanted to be special and to be loved.

The Doc answered the Kid's questions, but the Kid thought about his heroes as the Doc recited the textbook.

Eric, 65, was in the Kid's gang. They'd meet up and hang out most Sundays on the back pew, right-hand side, at St John's. Eric had once been a choirboy and knew the songs. The Kid was tone deaf.

Eric had been a diabetic since he was 29 and now couldn't see, so the Kid whispered the first line in Eric's ear and listened to him sing, and they'd laugh and get by. Eric couldn't move too well, as he had had both his legs taken off below the knee to stop the diabetic gangrene from spreading. But he moved well enough to go to lunch with the Kid. The next day, Steve, who was also in the Kid's gang, phoned the Kid. About 20 years earlier, Steve had always caught a train with the Kid from East Grinstead. One summer's day, now long ago but forever frozen in Steve's head, the Kid noticed Steve was sweatin' and kinda stumblin'. Everyone thought Steve was drunk. Steve wasn't drunk; he was in the very early stages of multiple sclerosis.

So, the day after the Kid and Eric had lunch, Steve had phoned and said to the Kid, 'Me [in a wheelchair for twenty years] and Eric [blind and no legs below the knee] are worried about you.' The Kid cried.

The Kid parked his thoughts and noticed the Doc was still speaking '. . . making great advances in hormone treatment and radiotherapy . . .' The Kid, who had done a bit of reading, suddenly realised he was in the middle of an academic-proprietary-high-ground-at-least-getta-knighthood-prostate-slash-burn-or-poison range war. The NHS, led by the Marsden, was on the poison and burn side. While the private London Clinic, driven by Roger Kirby (*Small Gland, Big Problem*) was big on the slash. The Kid laughed.

The Kid was happy to be with the Doc. As Stephen Stills said, 'Love the one you're with.' And as every cowboy knows, you gotta put yourself on one side or the other in a range war. Otherwise, you're definitely gonna die and the Kid didn't wanna die just yet.

So it's back to the hormone therapy and another visit on 14 December and maybe in January it'll be a bit of the state-of-the-art radiotherapy IMRT burn.

As the Kid strode back to his bike in the sun, he smiled 'cause he'd see Eric on Sunday and drop in on Steve on Monday and he could now tell them both not to worry.

The Kid
14 September 2005

So I now try to answer those five questions I posed back on 7 September 2005:

1. Is the cancer still confined to the prostate?
2. Has it migrated to other reproductive organs near the prostate?

3.   Has it spread to the lymph nodes, nearby?
4.   Has it spread to the lymph nodes, distant?
5.   Has it travelled to the bones?

And the answers:

1.   Who knows?
2.   Probably.
3.   Maybe.
4.   Possibly.
5.   Hopefully not.

Well, obviously don't expect certainty. Don't worry, just get on with your life. My next appointment is on 14 December 2005. The doctor doesn't speak about starting the IMRT treatment in January and says my shoulder is nothing to worry about.

Then there is another point: if the doctor sees me as Mr T3aN1M0, how do other people see me? Am I now 'the bloke with cancer'? Is this a good thing or a bad thing?

These past few ramblings seem to me to reflect aspects of the three things you need to deal with if you've got a cancer.

- **First, the mechanics of your cancer:** at this point in time, the five questions above are my immediate concern.
- **Second, the external factors:** financial position, relationships and other stuff specific to you.
- **Third, the internal factors:** what is going on in your head?

They are, of course, all interlinked, mutually inclusive. Each will sometimes appear to be more relevant than the others; all will change over time as life unfurls.

Right now, I'm thinking about my relationships with other people and how others now see me. My route has been to tell the world about the cancer, not that the world is necessarily that interested (but it does seem bits of it are; from the bottom of my heart, thank you, bits). If you decide to keep it private, the internal factors will loom much larger; I suppose it's the typical Lady Macbeth syndrome, internalising stuff so it's in your shadow side – 'Out, damned spot!' I respect and admire people like that, but I'm not that strong or that detached, and it's not my way. I send emails.

Friday, 16 September 2005

I've been invited to the launch of a book called *The Lions* at the Grosvenor Hotel, Park Lane. Since rugby union went professional in 1995, it has been dragged kicking and screaming into the twenty-first century. It's not better than it was, it's not worse than it was, it's just different. The shop window is now part of the sporting entertainment world. Professional rugby is largely funded by Sky TV and provides product (good product) for both armchair watchers and live spectators alike. The employees, both playing and administrative, are able, competent and earning their livelihoods doing something they enjoy. They are professional and keen to be seen as such. Something has been gained and something lost; I don't know what it is, and actually, does it matter? For a tiny minority, yes; for most of us, no. The game has evolved since the first rugby international (between England and Scotland in 1871 – Scotland won by one point) and will continue to change. At that first international match, there were twenty players on each side, three umpires in striped shirts, using flags not whistles, and it was a punting game.

No points for a try, it just meant you could then try for a kick at goal. One of the umpires on that day, the Rev W.W. Ormonde, said, 'The objective of rugby football is to produce robust young men with active habits and manly sympathies.' Maybe something of that sentiment has trickled down through the decades.

What I do know for a fact is that if you want to fill 1,200 seats with paying guests for a rugby-union book launch, all you need to do is give those guests what they want, which is a decent meal, a bit of history and tradition, some heroes, a short wander down Amnesia Avenue and a joke or two.

The Lions is a team of the best players from England, Scotland, Wales and Ireland (north and south) which tours every three or four years to either Australia, New Zealand or South Africa. So, at the lunch, the heroes were, from New Zealand, former All Black captain Sean Fitzpatrick, a psychopath on the field, apparently, and the most charming man off it, but not as disarmingly charming as the former Australia captain and stand-off Michael Lynagh (whom I'd like my daughter to marry, although distressingly he's already married. Is that a problem these days?). From South Africa there was former Springbok captain Morne du Plessis, a shy, compassionate, able man (and son of a shy, compassionate, able man who captained the Springboks), who was also terrifying on the pitch. Why do all these ex-players/captains do such a good impression of Dr Jekyll and Mr Hyde, the sporting version?

And the Lions: from England, Billy Beaumont with whom, as with a Ronseal product, you get what you see, which will do very nicely for all of us. Big Gavin Hastings from Scotland, and from Wales the captain of the 1971 British Lions, who won the series against the All Blacks, John Dawes. Heroes all, and by now they have learned the script. More than what the doctor ordered. They were presented to us by former Scotland three-quarter, TV and radio pundit and renowned master of ceremonies Ian Robertson, who finally introduced the hero's hero, Willie John McBride, captain of Ireland and the British Lions. In the world that is rugby-union football, professional or amateur, only Colin Meads from New Zealand can lay claim to sit at the same table. Yet not even Colin Meads led a side unbeaten around South Africa, as Willie John did in 1974.

It was John Gainsford, one of the great Springbok centres of the 1960s – of any era, come to think of it – who said of the '74 Lions: 'They were mentally tougher, physically harder, superbly drilled and coached and disciplined and united. They were dedicated fellows who were trained to peak fitness and who were prepared like professionals and who were ready to die on the field for victory.' Spot on, John, we were.

Yet when we left the UK, we didn't sit at the back of the plane telling each other how wonderful we were. We knew we were good and the 1971 Lions had set a precedent in New Zealand, but we tried to stay cool and put such thoughts to the back of our minds. There were a lot of things we didn't really think about as we set off on the tour, like the fact that we could be used by the South African government as propaganda for the apartheid regime. I doubt any of the boys thought seriously about not going on the tour. Why should they? We were young, we were fit, we wanted to play the Springboks. And, yes, we were selfish.

I believed that it was pointless not to go. What would it have altered? The South African-born Peter Hain – now a Labour politician – was then a vociferous anti-apartheid campaigner and thought differently. Barry Newcombe, the rugby correspondent of the *Evening Standard*, took Peter and me out to lunch. It was all quite amicable. Peter asked me not to go, I refused and that was about the sum of it. Regrets? Not really. Did we, by beating the Springboks 3–1 in the Test series, give a morale boost to the black population? No. Forget all this guff about humiliating the Springboks to the point where a mockery was made of Afrikaaner claims to be some kind of master race. We didn't humiliate them; we simply beat them because we were better than they were.

When I was in South Africa, I made a conscious effort to discover for myself what it was like living under apartheid, for both whites and blacks. Rugby seemed to open doors for me that others couldn't go through. I met Helen Suzman, a lifelong anti-apartheid activist, who retired in 1974 as the Liberal Progressive Party's sole member of parliament. A wonderful woman. She was once accused by a minister of asking questions in parliament that embarrassed South Africa. Her reply? 'It is not my questions that embarrass South Africa, it is your answers.' I also spent a day at the University of the Western Cape talking with students about apartheid and listening to their take on it. Why did I do it? It wasn't because I felt guilty; I didn't. I just wanted to learn more. I also went to and spoke at a debate at Wits University.

Did I learn anything? Who knows? Maybe I did, although not always in the ways I would've liked. We had two games against non-white sides. The first was against the Proteas (the Cape Coloured side), although they were then called the South Africa Rugby Federation XV. We won 37–6 and it was probably the only time in my career I was glad the pitch was ringed with armed police. You could feel the anger from the supporters; the atmosphere at that game was heavy with resentment.

The second game, in East London against the Leopards, was completely different: it was carnival time. They were a Zulu/Xhosa team, and even though we won easily, 56–10, they had some talent. Morgan Cushe, for example, a flanker, who, had he been born a quarter of a century later, would have made a name for himself in world rugby. After the match, one of the black journalists asked me to come with him to see the real Africa in one of the townships outside Port Elizabeth. I think it was called Mdantsane. Some of the Leopards were there, and though they were surprised to see a white face, they couldn't have been kinder to me. I asked them if they'd like to come back to our hotel. The Leopard players laughed. 'Oh yeah! And the moment you leave town, then what happens?' Just guys trying to get by and lead a life in an impossible situation.

Of course, one of the main reasons we got such great results on that tour was our captain. Willie John is a living legend. You want the real deal, he's it. He was born just another scally from Ballymena, and he had a reputation for being big, Irish and difficult. When he was a young man he could apparently do a passable imitation at times of two planks that weren't particularly long. As an ex-player, he was not brilliant at selecting, managing or coaching, and he tried all of them. But as a player, as a leader of men, his chance came in 1974 as captain and so much more on the Lions tour to South Africa. He led 30 of us on a 22-match, 3-month tour into the heartland of South African rugby and brought us all out alive and undefeated.

Why did we all love Willie so much? Not because of his ability as a player – there are many great players in the history of the game. Not because of his ability as a leader – there are many great leaders in the history of the game. Not because he had twice been to South Africa with the

Lions before, in 1962 and 1968, and spoke from experience. (Although in the six Tests Willie John had played, do you know how many he'd won? None.) No, we loved Willie because he unreservedly loved all 30 of us.

Not just the Test team but all of us. If you get into the Test team, you are getting what you want; if you're in the Wednesday side – 'the dirt-trackers' – then within your terms of reference, even though you are part of one of the best teams in the world, you are failing. That's when the temptation is to go to the nearest bar, line up the beers and get horizontal. Willie John never let that happen, because he too had been a dirt-tracker once. He knew about disappointment, about rejection, about feeling unloved, and that's why he never let us feel any of those things in South Africa.

He couldn't put 30 of us in a team of 15. So what did he do? Well, it doesn't sound much some 33 years on, but at the time it made us feel like we'd just won the pools. It was early in the tour, at the dinner after we'd beaten Western Province in Cape Town on a Saturday. Already, it was clear that the squad was divided into 'goats' – the Saturday team – and us 'sheep', the midweek dirt-trackers. In his speech that evening, Willie asked his teammates to stand up. The goats stood up. We sheep wriggled in our uncomfortable seats. Willie again asked the team to stand up. We sheep stood up. Thirty of us were standing. We all looked at each other, eye to eye across a sea of those who could only sit. He wasn't going to let us slip away, he knew how we felt, and this was all he could do, the best he could do to let us know that he knew how it was for us sheep. We were one and would remain so until we trickled down the sink. The Springboks had no answer.

In the Third Test, in Port Elizabeth, where Phil Bennett inspired us to a victory that meant we were the first Lions team that century to win a series in South Africa, Willie made the team run over to us – us, the rags, the extras, the dirt-trackers, the also-rans – and made them applaud us. Again, it might not seem much, but we loved him and them for it. Willie cared about us then and would care about us forever. We were in his gang, no questions on either side. Show us the broken glass, Willie!

And then there was Syd Millar, the coach. Syd is now the chairman of the International Rugby Board, but back then he was another Ballymena boy – what do they put in the water over there? – and had been on the 1968 Lions tour to South Africa. Rumour had it he'd seen a fair few hospitals thanks to the local on-pitch hospitality. That's why he and Willie John made sure we wouldn't get pushed around this time.

As for what actually went on on the pitch, it's all been said before: played 22, won 21, drawn 1, lost 0; points for 729, points against 207. We won the Test series 3–0 and the Second Test scoreline of 28–9 was then the heaviest defeat in the Springboks' history. In the Third Test, we came close to thumping them by an even bigger margin. We failed by just three points – 26–9 – but there was plenty of the other kind of thumping going on nonetheless.

Clem Thomas, a former Lion himself and later a rugby correspondent, described it as 'the most violent Test I ever witnessed . . . I sat there in amazement as two massive fist fights broke out, one in each half.' This was when the infamous '99' call was said to have been used by the Lions. Legend has it that when Willie shouted '99', the team was to wade into the fray, all fists flying. It wasn't a feature of the midweek matches, but they were less physical than the Tests. The '99' call has been embellished down the years. It might have happened once or twice, but to hear some of the stories now, you'd think we were shouting '99' when we came down to breakfast and discovered they'd run out of orange juice.

Without question, though, it was Willie John's view that, while we were in South Africa to play rugby, we shouldn't shirk the physical stuff. If they tried to intimidate us out of the game, he said, we must take it and let the ref sort it out; but as there were no linesmen, CCTV or television cameras and the ref was a South African who had to live there after we had gone, we would only survive if we kept our hands down and individually took it. It is true to say the game is now a faster and more physical and, with the coming of professionalism and the use of cards, cameras and post-match citings, a much less violent game, which is, I suppose, a good thing. But Willie John drilled it into us that if one got involved, we all must get involved. In the past, Springbok tactics had been to provoke individual players into a fight and then give them the mother of all pastings. On this tour, if they wanted a fight, they would have to take us all on. Anyway, this is all now anachronistic macho stuff. The world has moved on, as has South Africa.

In that Third Test, the Springboks were not battered into submission but outplayed by Welsh footwork. Their 'hard man', the magnificently named Moaner van Heerden, lived up to his name in the second-half after the second of the big bust-ups. He left the field in a bit of a state. The story goes that after that Test, Dr Danie Craven, president of the South Africa Rugby Board, was so ashamed of his side's capitulation that as he presented the new caps with their Springbok blazers, he said, 'It hurts me to be giving you these, because you have not earned them.' I don't believe that story: the Doc loved his Boks.

I got to watch all the mayhem from the sidelines, along with the rest of the midweek team. See, being a dirt-tracker did have its advantages! It was a privilege just to be on the tour, and we returned home conquering heroes – all of us, not just the Test side. If we'd left not realising what a special group of players we were, we were aware of it on our return. We knew we had done something magnificent, but more than that, we had all become the closest of friends. And even now, more than 30 years later, I still regard the team as such. If you play rugby in the professional era, you get a livelihood; if you played for love in the amateur era, you got a life. However, we had a reunion in 2003, and if you want to see reasons not to play rugby, you could have done worse than to attend. It must have been painful to watch us descending the stairs at the Grosvenor Hotel. Our sole topics of conversation were arthroscopies, hip replacements, knee replacements and arthritis. But none of us would have missed that tour for the world. Whereas in '74 tour manager Alun Thomas would get annoyed because I'd never wear my blazer, now, over 30 years on, I wear it with pride. Got there eventually, Alun.

Time ticks on, and the Grim Reaper starts to gather us in: Alun Thomas, Choet Visser, our liaison man, and then Gordon Brown – 'Broon from Troon' – that Scottish giant of a second row, who never took a backward step on a rugby pitch and never took a backward step in confronting the cancer which finally took him in 2001. The night of the reunion, I remembered Gordon standing between his brothers in the same function room a few years earlier as he bid us farewell in his fearless, frank and funny way. You are still with us Broonie, and we with you.

Willie was there for Gordon until the end, and so it was no surprise to receive a phone call from him saying he had heard my news, he was in London on 16 September, would I come and join him at this book launch (which, incidentally, was sponsored by Price Waterhouse Coopers, the firm with whom, in another time zone, I'd taken my accountancy articles). So I'm in the drinks room before the meal, and they all know I've been diagnosed with cancer. Everyone is kind, they don't see a man with cancer and then me but the other way around. If there is a silver lining to this disease, it has been the love and concern that I have received. Part of me enjoys having cancer just for the spotlight. Am I such an attention seeker that I need a nasty disease to feel loved and appreciated? Shallow or what? The lunch is good, but the banter is better. The Lions of '74 – still roaring.

Saturday, 17 September 2005

Don't get the wrong idea here, I try not to live in the past, but the following evening I went to a pub in Central London for a 40-year reunion of the foundation students of the University of East Anglia, who started their courses in 1965. I actually didn't go to UEA until 1966, but I had somehow got onto the email list. It's strange, at school or college you, or at least I, always feel slightly deferential to those in the year or years above, even years later.

Anyway, UEA *circa* 1966–9, as anyone who was there at the time will tell you, was unquestionably the centre of the known universe. Now, 40 years on, we were smashed and battered but still standing – well, some of us. The definition of success, for me, was Ron Hecht, who was still alive and still nuts and has never worked a day in his life and is still in his own head, which must be a strange place to be – trapped with a young man shrieking quotations from Spengler. The reunion reminded me of a Joe Cocker concert I'd been to in Shepherd's Bush about five years earlier. The gas fitter from Sheffield looked bad, but not half so rough as the audience – a life of excess had left its mark.

So at the reunion, having been diagnosed with prostate cancer was no big deal. Robbie Richards had had something unpleasant for 12 years, and Liz Lloyd had something going on in her throat. We swapped tales of those no longer able to swap tales and drank their health. The surprising thing was that the women had held themselves together far better than the men (with the exception of Paul Dale, who out-Cliff-Richarded Cliff Richard). We men put it down to HRT and their unfulfilled lives, and then we carried on drinking. Cancer: no interest. Get over it or die.

On the other hand, the veteran scullers at TSS, like the guys at the Lions reunion, show love and concern, which I embrace and thank them for from the bottom of my heart. However, you've got to ask the question, why? Well, in part it's the best of all possible reasons: because they are concerned human beings, and, of course, I'm great and deserve it. But maybe it's not just to do with me; maybe they are concerned for themselves. Maybe if I, a fit, non-smoking man with no previous medical form and long-living antecedents, can get it, then so can they. Maybe they are scared.

It's strange, but I'm not scared, I want to help them and tell them that it's OK. That they are going to be OK.

Tuesday, 20 September 2005

Am I always so strong? I've taken a week out with my two girls before they go back to uni, on a Mark Warner end-of-the-Mediterranean-sun-season cheapo in Greece. Elisabeth has stayed at home looking after Mouse and recovering from the exertions of ten days' sightseeing in

Rome with a group from St John's, our local church. Much as I love them, I managed to get out of that one.

I love my girls and they, in part perhaps because of this disease, seem willing to show they love me. What more can a parent want? We've got over the 24 June stage – 'It's unequivocal. You've got prostate cancer,' and all the baggage that goes with that – and reached the 'Fetch me the remote, Clouds,' 'Get it yourself,' stage. Back to normal, as we were before 4 June. Almost.

At the moment, I'm thinking about the external factors, and in particular relationships with friends and family.

There seems to be one constant piece of advice, whether written or spoken, from fellow sufferers of any sort of cancer, although crucially those giving it have usually moved on from the state of uncertainty that I am still wallowing in. (That state, to remind myself rather than you, is that I have been diagnosed with locally advanced prostate cancer and am being given hormone treatment. This seems to be working, but are we shutting the stable door after the horse has escaped? With a Gleason 7 and an opening PSA 133, it is possible that the awareness in my right arm is due to androgen-independent cancer cells entering the lymphatic system, growing in the lymph nodes under my arm and spreading into my right upper arm, the humerus. Or is it just a bit of arthritis? In due course, I will find out.) That constant piece of advice is: 'Be positive. If there is to be a way through this, a positive attitude is required.' Usually with the added courageous doxology, 'I/We are going to fight this and I/we are going to win.' But you've got to at least ask the question, is that right? Isn't the course of what will happen dependent on that first aspect, the mechanics of the disease, and where you are within that framework of medical mechanical torture and all the associated uncertainty? Sure, I believe in giving self-delusion a go, but I'm sufficiently rational to acknowledge the inevitable. Dying from cancer isn't losing. It's just dying from cancer, and we've all got to die of something at some time.

Maybe if my cancer has metastasised into my humerus (great name) and I do move into the terminal stage, usually defined as a life expectancy of six months or less, I will see things differently. But, hey, life is ultimately, for everyone, a terminal business.

Maybe it's just semantics (and here I am hopping about to the third aspect, what is going on in my head); perhaps my way of 'being positive' is what I would call embracing life, loving life, making the most of whatever is left, enjoying friends and family and the minutiae of stuff, like the clean white-linen tablecloth in front of me. Is this desperate? Well, yes, but so what? I am desperate, but I love and embrace life in all its colours and shapes and sizes. If this is being positive, then in spite of wherever I stand with regard to the medical position, I know I will be positive forever. There is also a side effect in embracing life or being positive or whatever you wish to call it, and that is it makes everything that is thrown at you easier to deal with and easier for others around you.

So I come back to the question I asked at the beginning of this section. Am I always so strong? Well, of course not. I'm just another person with a potentially nasty disease trying to get through it. Actually, it would be more honest if I rejigged the words in the last sentence to read: 'I'm just trying to get through it, another potentially nasty person with a disease.'

Paradoxically, I seem to be at my weakest when I am happiest. So I'm just lying there, early afternoon in the warm end-of-season Greek sunshine, catching the rays on the beach. Stef is somewhere out in the blue bay doing her

Royal Yachting Association Level 2 course. Beautiful, fun and funny Clouds is beside me; she sees I'm crying. I don't mean to cry. Why should I lumber her, burden her? Hey, aren't I the one who will embrace life forever?

'Why are you crying, Pop King?'

'Nothing, Clouds, it's nothing.'

She sits on the sunlounger and puts her arms round me and kisses me. 'You can tell me, Dad.' When she was born and the midwife passed her to me, she opened her eyes for the first time and she saw me and I saw her. We both love that story.

So I tell Clouds why I am crying. As I am, for the first time, crying unashamedly for myself.

I was just thinking, Clouds, when my dad died, he was cremated in Cheltenham and the service was full of 'For Those in Peril on the Sea'-type hymns, as he had spent 50 years or more at sea as a chief engineer, most of the time with the Cunard Line. You know, Clouds, you can actually say your granddad worked for Cunard.

My parents separated when I was seven, the youngest of five. We left Liverpool, the five of us brought up by my wonderful mum in Bristol. When we kids had all taken our lives elsewhere, my mum and dad tried to live together in Winchcombe; it didn't work – mum was too independent – and they separated again.

My dad had always been the apple of his mother Hope Ripley's eye, his three elder sisters never stood a chance. He got lucky. Like his sisters, he went into service. He was a valet, but the man he worked for saw he was a bright boy and paid for his education, and he went to Toxteth Technical College, where he trained as a marine engineer. After the cremation, before you were born, me and my brother and three sisters went to his parents' grave in Lincolnshire, and his ashes were buried with his mother and father; my brother and sisters let me write the inscription for the headstone: 'George Alwynne Ripley 1902–1984 Home Safe to Harbour'.

When Mum, Nana, died (she lived with us for the last eight years of her life), and as you know, Clouds, she was loved by her children and in-laws and grandchildren and great-grandchildren and you, she was cremated; she didn't want to be buried as in Liverpool during the war a bomb from an air raid had hit the graveyard next to where we were living in Woolton and disinterred the corpses. She didn't like what she saw and as a result didn't want to be buried. So she was cremated, and some of her ashes were thrown over the Wash Pool on Cleeve Hill, because she wanted her spirit to be in the hills in the Cotswolds, my sister Eileen took some and the rest were interred in her grave at St John's. Graham Paddick, our vicar, is very flexible. Mum agreed to this before she died, just to make me happy, so I could have somewhere to go to be with her. Pointless, I know, because she is actually always with us in our hearts. Mum always lived her life to make us happy. Again, my brother and sisters let me write the inscription for the headstone: 'Jessie Ripley 1908–2000 Surrounded by Love'.

'So why were you crying, Pop King?'

'Because I'm a silly old man and I wonder who's going to write the inscription for my headstone.'

I've hardly noticed, but the warm onshore wind has got up. Stef bounces back across the beach full of spray and life and laughing.

'Scary or what? I did more swimming than sailing. As the wind came up, the boat started to really fly, it was going so fast that I sped past the outer marker buoy, did you see? And then I was frightened to go about because I knew I'd capsize and the sharks might get me.'

'Stef, there are no sharks in Kalamata Bay.'

'There might be.'

'Stef, this is a Mark Warner holiday. No one, as far as I know, has ever been eaten by a shark on a Mark Warner holiday. I don't believe there has ever been a shark attack in Kalamata Bay or in Greece or in the Mediterranean. If you want to worry, worry about going past the outer marker buoy not about sharks.'

'Yes, Dad, but you don't know for certain. There might be sharks.'

'Yes, Stef, if you like, there might be sharks.'

We pick up our beach towels, go to the beach bar and each have a beach-boy iced coffee with an extra scoop of vanilla ice cream; and the sun is warm on our faces.

Wednesday, 21 September 2005

It's about three months since I was diagnosed with cancer, and I suppose we must be moving today into and out of some other zodiac signs; astrologically, Cancer is now well past. I don't know how I've changed, but I seem to have some antennae that pick up on other members of the Cancer Club and encourage them to talk to me. I have no problem, in fact possibly the opposite, letting people know about the fact I have been diagnosed with cancer, but there is a time and place for shutting up and getting on with living and not becoming a single-issue drone. The lady who sat next to me at lunch a couple of months ago and said, 'Oh no, not another old man droning on about his illnesses,' was not wrong. Everybody has issues, everybody has stuff to deal with. If I want to think about cancer stuff, I'll do it here in this record I'm keeping and not lumber or bore other people on holiday with my trivial concerns. At least that was the plan.

So all three of us are having a drink before dinner in the bar just up from the beach, with its wooden chairs and tables facing the sweep of the moonlit, still bay. The bar is full and we have sat down in the last three empty chairs, opposite Eileen, a few years older than me, and her husband. Stef has noticed Ray before because not only is he a brilliant windsurfer but if he is not windsurfing, he is playing tennis, and later that week he finished up winning the veteran tennis cup. Ray must be late 60s and is shy but does a more than just passable impression of Action Man. Eileen is fun and not shy and within thirty seconds tells us that she used to be like Ray until five years ago she was diagnosed with colon cancer.

Maybe I encourage her to talk about it more than I should, but I ask her lots of questions. I'm sympathetic – who wouldn't be? – but I also see a bit of me that I'm not too sure I like. I feel like a card player who is holding the ace of trumps. Sure, I'm going to play it. The question is when. Eileen tells me, I listen. Then, just before we get up for dinner, I tell her that I have recently been diagnosed with prostate cancer. She smiles. I smile. We are in the Club together. We go in to dinner. We remain friends but never talk about cancer again. We are partners, we are equal, we both know how it is without saying anything.

Tuesday, 27 September 2005

This is a busy day. Up at 7.30, take Marcus to Lingfield station so he can catch the train to work. The girls went back to uni yesterday, so the house is quiet. Torben, brown and curled up on his blanket by the stove, looks fed up. He knows he'll just have to wait for Elisabeth to take him for his walk.

Breakfast. I used to have big fry-ups, lots of bacon, eggs

and wedges of butter on the toast; now it's muesli, wedges of butter on the toast and coffee (and still the occasional fry-up).

In East Surrey Hospital in Holmwood Ward, Section C, Bed 4, one of the heart patients, a youngish man in Bed 5, had a packet of cigarettes on his table, and periodically he went outside for a quick fag. Saint Shrilla, on her morning round, looked at him, looked at the cigarettes and said, 'You're having an angiogram this afternoon, do you think that's sensible?'

'It's my little treat.'

Is breakfast my little treat? When the stimulus for prostate cancer is found (as smoking has been found to cause heart disease and lung cancer), I'm sure it will be to do with diet and saturated fats.

I go to Lingfield Surgery for 8.30. Lynne checks my INR: stable at 2.4, still on 14 mg of warfarin. Besides preventing, by thinning my blood, another embolism, the only other effect seems to be that my varicose veins have disappeared. A further benefit is having a chat with Lynne. She also gives me my 28-day shot of Zoladex. I ask her if we should change to a 12-week shot, and she says that we can but as I seem to be doing well with things as they are, why change? Smart lady, Lynne.

So what effects to date have three months of this luteinising hormone-releasing hormone (LHRH) coupled with the initial 30-day oral course of low-dose Casodex had on me?

Well, it's obviously killed off some of the prostate-cancer cells (the death of these cells is sometimes referred to as apoptosis) and stopped others from splitting and growing. Some cells are androgen-independent, and these will be unaffected and keep on growing. Hormone therapy will not cure prostate cancer, but in my case it does seem to be working. How do I know this? Because the PSA test taken on 5 September was 1.1 and because when the bouncy prof did a DRE on 17 August, it was 'not that impressive'.

However, it's a Faustian pact, because this potential deferment of the end of the piece of string comes at a price. I don't seem to need to shave every day any more, but on the other hand, my hair, which was thinning rapidly, seems to be thicker. I do seem to be thickening at the waist; there's been no weight change – still about 115 kg – but a loss of muscle. I don't seem to be developing breasts. Neither, to date, have I had hot flushes. Elisabeth is going through the menopause; there's obviously no fun in hot flushes. I urinate usually about once during the night and don't seem to have problems with stream or urgency. My testicles have shrunk and so, sometimes, has my penis, especially when I sit down on the toilet. I last ejaculated in July. I get periodic erections but have no libido.

I'll come back to diet, exercise and impotence later.

After the appointment, Elisabeth drops me off at the station, cheapo travel card and take the 9.14 to Victoria. I went back to university seven years ago when I was fifty, a middle-aged self-indulgent gift to myself, to try to get better at rowing and trial for the Cambridge blue boat and, almost incidentally, do an MPhil. My dissertation was on considering the value of an accounting asset at an arbitrary accounting date and the allocation of profit across adjacent accounting periods where the asset is contracts of employment. Exciting or what? But that's what I do, and happily.

After UEA and following my articles with Price Waterhouse in the City and a year doing a postgrad at LSE, I worked in finance companies for about 25 years. Anyway, after Cambridge I wanted to work for myself: interim management, consultancy, non-executive directorships, some quoted companies, some private, some paid work, some not paid, some start-ups, some salvage – whatever interested me and was available. I also like teaching numbers, finance and writing. My most recent tome was *Forfaiting for Exporters*. Catchy.

So today I have an appointment at eleven o'clock to meet Darren Rawcliffe, mid-30s rising whizz-kid at Grosvenor Estates, to see if I can give him some one-to-one tutoring. (I specialised in financial training in property companies.) We immediately don't click. He's on his way to Planet Mercury, the stratosphere, and knows everything already; I'm possibly heading for the morgue and don't want to spend potentially limited time with people I don't want to be with. We are both smart enough to recognise this and knock it on the head. Sometimes things work, sometimes they don't. Darren and I are of the same opinion. Move on. I'm meeting former England player Marcus Rose for lunch. I wait in the Grosvenor Estates foyer and the very nice receptionist makes me a cup of coffee.

Marcus bounds in through the door. Marcus, 48, is a bit like Darren 10 years on, already on Planet Mercury. We played rugby together for England and Rosslyn Park. Marcus was always a top-class ball player and excelled at any sport he turned his hand to. Me, I was just big and could run quick. Our paths never really crossed after Marcus left Rosslyn Park, but when they did, we enjoyed each other's company.

About ten years ago, November time, Marcus had been in a cinema with his wife and a couple of friends, watching a film he didn't want to see, when he became aware that although he didn't want to see the film, he couldn't actually hear the soundtrack. Probably something trivial. It wasn't. Unbeknown to him, he had a brain tumour. Christmas, New Year, pain, headaches and increasing loss of hearing and balance. The good news was that the tumour was probably benign, not cancerous. But they wouldn't know till the pathologist looked at cells from it under the microscope. Left to grow in the confinement of his skull, the tumour would press against the brain, and he was just in the foothills of the symptoms. He needed to have it removed. Some skilled skull opener did the job. Marcus recovered. It's strange that those two words should cover such a period of anxiety and fear in his life.

Before the operation, some of his friends had sent a large cheque to the Atkinson Morley Hospital with a note to say that they would appreciate it very much if at the same time as the surgeon was doing his wonderful work, he could also give Marcus a personality transplant.

Since he found out I have prostate cancer, he has been bothering me. We have a good lunch. I cry at some stage. He won't let me share the bill. We kiss each other goodbye. Kissing Marcus Rose – blimey, if A.K. Rodgers, old friend and Cambridge rugby coach, finds out, I'll be drummed right out of the Brownies. I seem to be kissing a lot these days. I like it. I like Marcus.

Bond Street, Tube to Liverpool Street. I'm five minutes late for a board meeting at DHSM at three. DHSM had been a syndicate management agency at Lloyd's of London, but its five syndicates had ceased to underwrite in 1999, and it is now in run-off. I am a consultant and non-exec director helping in that process of putting it to sleep. At five, I go round the corner to another board meeting of an insurance underwriting company called Lead Yacht Ltd. This is a working entity and working well. I wrote to Peter Sangster, Lead Yacht's chairman (whom I'd known for a long time; sadly, his wife had recently died of a heart condition), after I was diagnosed as prostate-cancer positive, as I did to all the chairmen of the companies I was involved with, offering my resignation. He wrote back and said I'd have to come up with a better reason for leaving. Allan and Vlad, who, with Peter, own the company, seem happy to have me around.

At 6.30, I get back on the Central Line to go to the Lansdowne Club just off Berkeley Square, where I meet Jonathan Shingleton.

Besides writing those letters to various chairmen, I had resolved to do three things, and maybe more. First, because I felt so grateful to the NHS – well, not so much the NHS as the people who worked for them – I wanted to say thank you, do something to help. Well, all I do is numbers, so I resolved to apply for a non-exec post at the NHS trust nearest to me if such a position became available. I had been a non-exec in a health trust in the mid-'90s. This is a labour of love. The Government, the patients, the employees, grieving relatives, who would, understandably, externalise their grief by attending the public board meetings, were all looking for a scapegoat, and who better than the trust's board of directors – the suits. It's a form of public stocks for the twenty-first century. Three years of this at a daily rate, after tax and national insurance, of about £8 a day had been enough. It wasn't the money.

Companies are driven by the profit motive. Revenue less expenses, and the balance – net of tax – is the potential return to the owner. A hospital's revenue is the unquantifiable sum of the patients' well-being. The costs are the sum allocated by the Government. At some stage, someone has to make a decision about how much a human life is worth. Impossible. This obviously has considerable resonance for me at the moment: will I get the IMRT treatment in January or will it be deferred or cancelled as part of a hospital budgeting exercise? Then there's the new foundation trusts and 'patient choice'. My understanding is that patients do not pay (yet) but will be offered a choice of hospitals, often including a private option, for their treatment. The hospital will then be paid by the Government for the individual treatments delivered. Will this work? One thing's for sure: being a non-exec on a trust board will make being put in the medieval stocks seem mild by comparison.

As they say, someone's got to do it. So I've applied for a non-exec position on the Bromley NHS Trust board. Maybe my application will get lost – this is the NHS! Maybe I won't make the shortlist, maybe they'll find someone better. Maybe they'll pick up my hat and then maybe I can try to do my best. I spend time filling in the massively politically correct public-service form, and although I'm the usual white, middle-aged, middle-class male who applies for this sort of position, I bet none of the other applicants ticks the disability box and writes, 'Currently being treated for a pulmonary embolism and just diagnosed with prostate cancer.'

Second, I decided to write this. Is this therapy? Possibly. It certainly isn't original, but it seems a good idea to keep some sort of record, and I'm enjoying it. I am still undecided what, if anything, to do with it.

Third, Doug – you remember, Doug from Tideway Scullers, 10 years ago aged 45, annual company medical, PSA increased to 7, DRE uncertain, Gleason score 6, followed by a radical prostatectomy – had given me the book *Small Gland, Big Problem*, his best wishes and the most recent copy of the quarterly magazine from the Prostate Research Campaign UK charity, the sort of specialist publication that will probably feature on *Have I Got News for You* one day. Amongst the many articles, tucked away on an inside page, was a short paragraph relating that in order to raise funds for the charity, Jonathan Shingleton was looking to fill a yacht with prostate-cancer sailors to compete in the 2005 Atlantic Rally for Cruisers, a race for cruising yachts from the Canaries to St Lucia: bizarre but interesting enough to get involved.

I thought, as I at least qualified on medical grounds, I'd send Mr Shingleton an email. When we meet up, he says the boat, an Oyster 47 called *Kindness* (the surname of the doctor who discovered the lump in his prostate and referred him to a specialist), already has a crew for the race, but if I want it, there is a berth from Plymouth to the Canaries, leaving on 10 October. Across the Bay of Biscay in late October? I ask if I can just do the Cadiz to Canaries leg, about 800 miles, about 5 days' sailing.

In an earlier life, some 20 years ago, I took a year-long land-based yachtmaster's course, and at the end of the course, in May, some of us hired a Sun Kiss 40 out of Falmouth and sailed to the Scilly Isles, back to Jersey, then in and out of the north Brittany coast, down to Cape Finisterre and then back to Plymouth. Long periods of boredom interspersed with periodic brown-trouser stuff, but fun. I then sailed with Tim Cowell, an old rugby friend of mine who had been on the unbeaten England tour to South Africa in 1972. It was Tim who was there with his wife Maria when Mike called me over on 24 June. He has a Bavaria 30 and we used to sail a bit in that out of Hayling Island Sailing Club.

However, my big sailing deal was being a halyard bouncer in a Swann Racing series, about ten years ago. There are about 20 in a big-boat racing crew: meatheads on the grinders, owners and tossers in the rear and nits, snowboarders and mountain-bike riders on the foredeck. All a halyard bouncer does is this: as the boat swings round the windward buoy, in that static instant, you've got to get the kite up before it fills with wind and weight. Grinders are too slow, so you need two people bouncing the halyard, one tall and strong – obviously me – and one small and strong – that was a guy called Mike. Get it right, and it's easy and takes fractions of a second. That's all you do, other than sitting on the windward side eating pies. Very appropriate in our case, since our boat, *Taipan of Wales*, was owned by Stan the Pie. He and his brothers had sold their business in Wales, Brain's Pies, after which Stan indulged himself by sailing big boats, while his brother Peter got involved with Cardiff Rugby Club. Difficult to say which brother had the most fun – or which one got the worst deal.

Anyway, Stan had about three professional crew and a bunch of mates from Merthyr and a bunch of ex-rugby players. It worked well. In these races, the best fun was not to be had when one of the professional crew was helming, since this was their job and if they bent the boat, they'd be out of a job. On the other hand, there was one occasion when Stan, always with an eye for the main chance, invited a French woman who had just done one of those big single-handed races to helm in one of the Juan Carlos series in Majorca. In a big afternoon triangle race, everything is in the start. It's dangerous, and it's the helm who risks everything who wins. She really didn't care about the boat; it was really scary bully-boy tactics (well, bully-girl, actually). Sitting on the side, I even dropped my pie as it looked as if we were about to cream the host's boat. Not much made the colour drain from Stan's face. She did. But we made it bang across the line in pole position. Juan Carlos waved. She never helmed again – Stan isn't a businessman for nothing – but us pie eaters sitting on the side waiting for our nanosecond of activity loved it.

I don't bore Jonathan with that stuff. He was diagnosed 7 years ago, aged 51 – raised PSA level but higher than usual, about 30. He went to Roger Kirby and was put on a course of hormones prior to radiotherapy. He reacted badly to the hormones quite quickly, with severe hot flushes, but worse, he went yellow, as his liver also reacted badly. He was taken off the hormones and immediately given a six-week radiotherapy course. It seemed to work, and there were no unusual urinary problems or potency problems. Although he is, when we speak, having a PSA bounce, up to 4. Once you're a member of the Club, you're always a member.

We get on well and arrange that I will meet the boat in Cadiz harbour, either late on 21 October or early the next morning, as we are due to leave on the afternoon of 22 October.

I catch the 8.23 home from Victoria. A busy day indeed.

Wednesday, 28 September 2005

Up at 5.30, slice of toast for me and one for Torben. On the bike to get to Chiswick at 6.45 to meet my friend Rak for a pairs outing. I'm on stroke side, he's on bow. We intend to enter for the Pairs Head race on 15 October, Hammersmith to Chiswick. I want to see how we go. No, I want to see how I go.

Rowing on the Thames, particularly in the early autumn as the dawn comes up, is special. You can't believe you are in central London. We always start against the current; today, it's upstream towards Richmond, the first half-weir on the tidal Thames. It's the last knockings of an ebbing low tide and sunny and just after the autumnal equinox, so the water is really low. Because of the shape of the Thames, the current flows out for just over seven hours and in for about five. So just on a probability basis, we usually row upstream first rather than down to Putney or, more usually, Hammersmith. Although each of us has separately won medals in the world veteran championships, we have never won much together. But we are both prepared to turn up on time, and that, it seems to me, is the prime requirement in rowing: to turn up.

I'd never turned up anywhere to row until the early 1990s. After my brief flirtation with rowing in the *Superstars* TV competition, my interest had cooled. It was my old England teammate Roger Uttley who reignited my passion. Blimey, I'd never have thought that one day I would write those words in the same sentence: 'Roger Uttley reignited my passion.' Quick, call the men in white coats . . .

We had played together in a charity rugby match and Roger – a great pal who has been a physical education teacher at Harrow School since about 1932, is a former England Rugby Coach and had always been a wonderful ball-player – noticed that I was puffing a bit. So after the game he suggested I put my name down for an indoor-rowing competition, in which he was already entered, at Henley Management College the following week. So we went along and competed in the veterans category, which involved rowing 2,500 m as fast as possible. Roger came first and I was second. That was it – I had the rowing bug (well, the indoor-rowing bug).

I bought myself a Concept II rowing machine and began training hard at home. Midlife crisis? Maybe, but do you know how humiliating it is to lose to Big Rog? The only thing I ever had over him was I'd always been fitter than him. A few months later, I entered myself in the British Indoor Rowing Championships and won the 40–44 age category, rowing 2,500 m in 7 min. 53.6 sec. I retained the title for the next few years (in 1995, the official distance was reduced from 2,500 to 2,000 m) but still had no real desire to swap indoor rowing for outdoor. It was warm indoors, and I didn't get wet. I used to go to the Henley Regatta on corporate junkets, and I'd never actually watch the rowing. I'd be aware it was going on, but I'd be with everyone else in the tent with my back to it. Corporate hospitality, dontcha love it? I did.

Then, in about 1996, I saw an advert in my local paper, the *East Grinstead Courier*, in which a local rowing club invited veterans to come down and row. No previous experience required. After a few basic coaching sessions with the help of Ian Wilson, head honcho of Concept II, ex-international oarsman and general mayhem-maker, I was persuaded by him to compete in the Trent Head of the River Sculling Race. Presumably I was the comic turn; I'd never sculled before in my life. But Ian found me a boat and put me in it. Within seconds, I'd put myself out of it. I think I fell in three times before my race actually started. When it did, I fell in twice more, and I eventually finished just as it was getting dark.

But I wasn't disheartened. Who cared if I came last? I saw it as a challenge to improve. I forked out for my own boat and joined a club on the Thames called the Tideway Scullers. There, a wonderful chap called Alec Hodges taught me how to scull properly, and instead of finishing last in races, I began to win the odd one or two. Rowing gradually took over my life.

There had been a moment back in June 2005, in hospital, when I'd thought I would never, could never, row again. So to be on the Thames now, with the sun rising on a crisp autumn morning, is just heavenly. I don't push myself, and Rak seems OK with that. As yet, I don't know where I am physically; just doing it is a start. We settle into a familiar pyramid routine (a pyramid session is one in which you alternate hard work with easy going). Rak, at bow, steers, keeps a lookout and rows; I just row. In sweep rowing (you have one oar), as in sculling (two oars each), you face the wrong way to go forwards. The only other sports in which you face backwards to go forwards are backstroke swimming, high jump (provided you are flopping) and tug of war – maybe some diving or dressage could make the cut. I've always been surprised that the tug of war has never had a revival: stick it in the Olympics – brilliant TV. A bunch of sumo wrestlers from Japan against a WWF team representing the USA for a gold medal has got to be televisually workable. Sport is now about entertainment as well as two old men paddling a boat in the early morning on the Thames.

From the changeover point at Chiswick, we keep to the left-hand bank on the ebb, which, of course, as we are facing backwards, is on our right-hand side. We turn round near Syon House at the changeover point just after the barges. Well warmed up, we take off our sweatshirts to row the 5 km back in one stretch in the centre of the stream. There is a magic in rowing that you either feel or you don't. We sit at backstops – legs flat with the sliding seat fully extended on the back of the slide, backs straight, no tension, balancing the static boat, blades square in the water. We don't say anything. I push the handle down, Rak follows me, hands away, turn the blade parallel to the water by rolling the shaft with my right hand, move up the slide slowly, roll the blade with my right hand so it's square to the water again and let the blade fall into the water; arms extended, push away with my feet gently, the boat moves forward. Legs extended, finish the stroke off by pulling with my arms round the turn, and repeat. As the boat starts to flow, repeat the action, shoulders relaxed, lengthen out the stroke, don't rip the water. As the boat picks up the rhythm, remember at frontstops, when your legs are compressed before you push away with the legs, to use the arms just to connect the blade with the water. Let the momentum of your body do the work. 'Leave it out there.'

We all do dumb stuff. I suppose that's what makes life the opposite of arid. But slinging in a good job to try to get in the Cambridge blue boat was an odd thing to do. There I was, nearly 50, with a comfortable life, about to do that odd thing. Thanks to some dealings with Lloyd's of London, which thankfully didn't bankrupt me, and a good job with a trade finance house, I had money. Now, I could do one of two things with the money: I could buy 'stuff' (but I had enough stuff, and I've never been into material possessions to any great degree); or I could buy my life back. I decided to do the latter.

What did I love doing? I asked myself. Rowing. Where can I row? Cambridge. So I went up to Cambridge to do a Master of Philosophy degree. Or rather I went up to Cambridge to try to become the oldest person to row in the Boat Race.

So, in September 1997, I swapped living in my comfortable house for a third-floor bedsit at Hughes Hall graduate college overlooking Fenner's cricket ground. At the end of the month, I turned up at the Goldie Boathouse for a trial, along with fifty others who dreamt of being interviewed live on *Grandstand* in six months' time. I knew that my weakness would be my lack of outdoor rowing experience. Most of the other trialists had been rowing since school and were far superior technically to me. They could move a boat efficiently. I would have to rely on brute strength and the wisdom of old age.

Strength is probably the last thing you lose with age but flexibility is the first. I came pretty well last in most of the flexibility tests, but fortunately a lot of emphasis was placed on work done on a Concept II rowing machine: 2,000 m as quick as you can. I'm a natural indoor rower – just under 2 m tall, 250 lb, a slow-beating heart, big lungs and a small brain. I'd waited for this moment. I was pretty well rubbish at everything else, but I could do this. I was on the machine looking through the big glass doors of the boathouse as the sun filtered across the Cam. Beyond Midsummer Common, I could see the spires of Jesus College. It was my moment. Then coach Ian Dryden walked over and adjusted the resistance of the rowing machine from level 10, the hardest, to level 5, mid-range. I stared at Ian. 'That's what we all do it on,' he said. All my training had been at resistance 10. I'd altered my life to be sitting there and suddenly the carpet had been pulled from under me.

What was the problem? Rowing at level 5 means the rower has to increase his stroke rate (his number of strokes per minute) from not much to lots to compensate for the reduced resistance. I was a strong rower but not a cardiovascular one. I'd be knackered! I got up and walked around the gym. I knew you never say anything, you just get on with it, because that's the way it is. Level 5 it was. I'd never done it at 5. Harry Mahon, another coach, knew; he smiled at me and said nothing. Unknown land. One shot, my best shot. I went through the first 1,000 m too fast – just under 3 min., but it felt easy – let it slip up a bit, not too much, and then held on for 6 min. 5 sec., the best I'd ever pulled. I said nothing. Harry smiled at me. Third fastest of the day – I was in.

A squad of about 40 was selected and that's when the fun really began: 4 gym sessions each week at 6.30 a.m. and 15 miles daily on the River Ouse in the afternoons and at weekends. Friday was a day off. Bless you, Harry. The day I turned 50, 1 December 1997, was a Monday. But

I loved the training, and I loved the chat among the squad. I'd forgotten what it was like to be 20. Sitting listening to their conversations, I realised they had worse problems than me: women, insecurity, naivety, endless youthful enthusiasm. I was just the old bloke in the corner content in my own skin. But the best thing was that they tolerated me, didn't seem to mind me being there and treated me as just another member of the squad, even though I was old enough to be their father.

I came home every Friday – you know what it's like, being a student, you return home every couple of weeks to get your washing done and eat something other than a Pot Noodle – and there I would be, in my pyjamas at quarter to eight in the evening. Marcus, who was then 16, would look at me and, with a shake of his head, say, 'Dad, you're so sad.' Elisabeth kindly indulged my self-indulgence.

I didn't see much of Harry after the September trials. Harry, about my age, was the finishing coach and really came centre stage in the last month or so before the Boat Race, so the little time he had was mainly spent with the potential blue-boat crew – that's what he was paid for, after all. In the third week in December, the rest of the university had gone home for Christmas and the rowing squad and coaches were the only ones left. It was a merciless day on the Ouse at Ely, with the cathedral in view, a strong easterly wind blowing the snow flurries all the way from the end of the world and lumping up the water. We had to row 22 km in a quad, me and my crew all knowing we were probably the ones who wouldn't make the final Boat Race squad. Numb hands, numb faces, numb minds. Then Harry appeared in a tin launch to offer words of gentle encouragement.

But Harry Mahon was like that. He was there for any rower who needed his help or wanted his advice. It didn't matter who they were: Olympic eights, world champions, novice schoolboys, even old men who should know better. Harry didn't care whom he helped, he just wanted people in boats to go faster. Harry. Kiwi, teak hard, didn't say much other than 'Leave it out there.' And even back then he must have known he had cancer. He never said much about it; even when everyone knew, he never really talked about it. He used the short time he had left on earth to fall in love and make people in boats go better.

I made the initial cut, and I survived the cull when the squad was reduced from 40 to 28, but when the final 18 was announced – enough for two boats plus a couple of spares – I was out. Dumped. Discarded. But with no regrets. I had given it my best shot. At least I was alive and fit and strong, and a heck of a better rower thanks to all my training. In 1998, I won the World Indoor Rowing Championship in the heavyweight 50–54 age category with a time of 6:07:7. It remains the British and world record for that age group. Cheers, Harry.

Back on the Thames with Rak in autumn 2005 and the boat starts to flow on the dying ebb tide as I leave it out there. Not many other boats about, the rate picks up with the boat and by the time we are back at Chiswick, our stroke rate per minute is up to 30. Rak goes to work after we arrange to go out again on Saturday morning, I take a shower. I'm glad no one else is about, as the sitting position seems to have shrunk my penis. The warm water helps things get back to OK. I have a cup of tea with Alec, the heart of Tideway Scullers. Aged 79, he is everyone's patriarch.

There is something great about exercise. You feel so good about yourself.

I'm on the M25 going home and the sun is up. I've always

liked bikes. The Triumph Rocket 3 is not a crouch and speed. Without a screen, in the sitting-up position, once you go faster than you should, the wind blows you so you can neither use the machine's power nor lose your licence. I'm on warfarin with an INR of 2.4; I hit the outside lane, open up the throttle and take the wind. I really should grow up.

Friday, 30 September 2005

A few days ago, I resolved to get to know more about this disease, about the first aspect, the mechanics of cancer. I visited Amazon.co.uk and found there are 248 titles about prostate cancer. I ordered eight books. If it's going to kill me, I want to know about it; if I get rid of it, I want to know what it is I'm getting rid of. If we have to share the future together, I want to know our modus operandi.

I decided to make myself responsible for myself as far as I can. Diet, exercise and sex are what I need to address, and I will. However, the first stop was to visit the dentist. I have had a tooth (left upper molar) periodically abscessing for the last five years, a constant source of infection with penicillin to knock it back. Two root canal fillings and a cap haven't resolved the problem. My dentist, Anne Gleason, sent me to a specialist surgeon, as warfarin and chronic infection are considerations. He gives me a consultation, tells me to have it out and then arranges to stick it in the bucket this morning at 8.30. With private dental treatment, you get what you pay for. John Tighe at the McIndoe Centre is good; in five minutes, he takes out the tooth and £250 from my wallet. I have no side effects, no after effects and no longer a constant source of infection in my head. Money well spent.

I have been put on the shortlist for the job at Bromley

NHS, and this afternoon I'll be interviewed by a panel of three. I arrive at the Princess Royal University Hospital an hour early to mooch about. The hospital was built in 2003, it's clean and you can tell the patients and staff seem proud of it. If I get selected, I'll be pleased to be a part of it.

It is a one-hour interview. There are five candidates, and I'm the last at 4.15. The interview panel (two men and one woman) is good, and they seem to know what they are looking for. I'm brutally honest about everything – no point being anything else. I'm not that well prepared, but I enjoy the process. I particularly enjoy the fact that they are obviously obliged, this being a public post answerable to the political-correctness police, to tick certain boxes and ask me certain questions. For example, the woman asks me, 'Do you consider this to have been a fair interview?' Cripes, life isn't fair, so why should this interview be any different?

The same well-intentioned lady – who I think may have been on a course – asks the question, 'If over a certain issue you disagreed with the majority of the board but you were in the minority, what would you do?' There is clearly a stock answer, but it probably isn't, 'Taking this question to its extreme, would I, even confronted by peer and institutional pressure, do something I knew was wrong? So, for example, if I had been a concentration-camp guard in Dachau would I have turned on the gas tap?' I didn't know the answer to my question. The chairman said it was OK because, as far as he knew, being a non-exec director of an NHS trust, I wouldn't actually be asked to kill anyone. We all smiled, but I couldn't help thinking that killing people is exactly the possible consequence of the decisions a budget-cutting non-executive director has to make.

I was naughty, but they were asking me their politically correct questions, so why shouldn't I ask the chairman of the board the usual old chestnut: 'If you had to describe your board as a vegetable, what vegetable would it be?' He stumbled about but kindly gave me an answer: 'A root vegetable, because this hospital has its roots in the local community.' This was OK, but not as good as the answer I got when I asked the same question, much to Clouds' embarrassment, of the headmaster of Epsom College at an open day for prospective parents. There was one crucial difference, though: at Epsom I was buying, and at Bromley NHS I was selling. After a long pause and some thought, the head, Tony Beedle, replied to the same stupid question, saying, 'It's a cabbage, because this school, too, has a big heart surrounded by many varied and different leaves, or students. All of whom we value.' Get the chequebook out, Elisabeth, Clouds is going to Epsom College sixth form.

The one thing the board doesn't ask me about is my prostate cancer, which surprises me.

Sunday, 2 October to Sunday, 9 October 2005

Elisabeth bought a sofa. It's huge and it's in the hall. I say, 'Why have you bought that huge sofa in the hall?' She says, 'It's OK, it's for the flat in Austria.'

'Don't they have sofas in Austria?'

'Yes, but not like this one.'

'How are we going to get that huge sofa from here to there?'

'In the car,' she says.

We have an old Range Rover, good for pulling out tree stumps in the garden and, when Clouds and Stef were younger, for pulling a horse box and for driving to Austria, which is why it has 150,000 miles on the clock and only lives because of Mr Tovey, a 75-year-old mechanical hero who keeps our rubbish cars running.

'How in the car?' I say.

Normally, at this stage, because this is actually fairly stupid, I'd go on, and Elisabeth, because she in her heart also knows it's stupid, would get very defensive. However, after 57 years of life and now 4 months of having been diagnosed with prostate cancer and being in touch with my feminine side, I get this inspiration: don't go on, but rather, 'cause this is going to happen anyway, agree to be stupid, fall in with it, accept it, get on with it, just go with the flow, try to make it work and with a smile on my face.

Life is now so easy. Why didn't I do this from the day I married Elisabeth? We get on great, and unbelievably, after much readjustment, we get the sodding sofa – both pieces and the associated cushions – into the car. Which is just as well, because on the 700-mile trip from Calais to Seefeld, it sluices down with rain. We take the 7.00 a.m. ferry from Dover on Sunday, 2 October, because lorries aren't allowed on the German autobahns on Sundays. A few minutes on the Net on Friday gets me a good deal. Experience has taught me to take the Calais–Dover route and see whether P&O, Sealink, Norfolkline or Hoverspeed offers the best rate.

About 10 hours' driving at 70 mph with a few stops gets the sofa to Austria. I've been making the same trip for 30 years now. The Tyrol has lots of things going for it, but for Elisabeth it's where her youth and her heart and her massive (both brothers about 2 m tall and 120 kg, and two sisters) extended family live. If I die, she will eventually go and live in her flat, which she/we are now turning into a two-bedroom Alpine palace. If I don't die, we will have somewhere really nice to stay.

Days in Seefeld fall into each other. It is a mountain lake paradise; everywhere you turn is the sound of music and more. We get up late and slowly have breakfast, read, walk, eat, see friends, and the sunny, warm autumn days slip by into each other.

On the Saturday night before we leave, we go and see one of those friends, Benno – about my age, ski teacher, yodeller, son of a Mexican American serviceman who, when his post-war tour of duty was done, probably didn't know he had left a son behind, although he found out later.

Benno is talented, he sings and smiles, all his life he has sung and smiled. This has got him into a lot of scrapes, shall we say. He has three marriages behind him, and his group, whom we go to see playing in the Hotel Eden, comprises him, one of his sons, Benjamin, from his second marriage, and Benjamin's new stepmother, who is Irish and five years younger than her stepson. Imear, from Cork, has the voice of an angel. Everything works. Elisabeth says Imear could sing like Peggy Lee and promises to send her a CD.

I've walked about three hours a day and read a lot, as I brought with me, as well as the sofa, the books about prostate cancer that had arrived just before we left, courtesy of Amazon. These are not medical textbooks, but rather guides written by oncologists and urologists to give punters like me who have some grade of the disease their take on the whole deal. There were, as I mentioned earlier, almost 250 titles available on Amazon.co.uk on this topic. As 1,000 American men are diagnosed with this disease every day, most (70 per cent) American men over 55 know their current PSA and something like $100 million is invested each year into research in the USA (about £4 million in the UK), there is greater awareness of and knowledge about prostate cancer in the States than in the UK. Consequently, most of these books are American; this doesn't matter too much as prostate cancer knows no political frontiers, although there would appear to be a certain ethnic/cultural/diet bias regarding its spread.

The relatively recent upsurge in interest, caused by increasing longevity and, since the 1980s, increased PSA testing, has led to changing attitudes towards the study of this disease. With this in mind, I bought one book which was printed in 1995 along with the 2003 edition to see if there was any change in emphasis.

My intention isn't to regurgitate everything I found out from these books (quite frankly, you would be far better advised to go and buy the source material, and there's a bibliography at the back of this book). What I wanted from them was to get a better grip on what exactly cancer is and, more specifically, prostate cancer and, even more specifically, my prostate cancer. I now do know more about this disease than when I was first diagnosed and will have more to say on what I learned later.

Tuesday, 11 October 2005

Today was going to be a good day. I knew this before it had even begun. Before the orange figures of my alarm danced and glowed. I knew this about mid-morning the previous day when I'd arranged to meet Paul Kimmage at one o'clock today near Eros at Piccadilly Circus. Paul had said, 'What is Eros?' So I knew it was going to be a good day. How can anyone not know what or where Eros is?

Is this a side effect of prostate cancer? Because now every day seems like a good day and it really doesn't seem to matter where I go or who I'm with or what I do. Have I – after 57 years of paying lip service to the idea – actually started living every day as if it were my last?

It seems like just a great place to be.

In fact, today did not begin too well. Before buying the

cheapo day travel card to catch the 11.44 from Lingfield station to Victoria, as I was competing in the Pairs Head this Saturday (Steve Jones, who knows nothing about rowing, suggested that the Pairs Head sounds like some sort of group sexual deviance – of no interest to me now, Steve), I decided to do a piece on the ergometer.

I hadn't been on the erg for a while. I'd give it a go. Just 3,000 m at 1 min. 48 sec. per 500 m, so that's 10 min. 48 sec. in total of huff and puff. This was not a hard session. Pre-pulmonary embolism, Casodex and Zoladex, it would not have been too taxing.

A thousand metres into the piece, and I just couldn't hold it, couldn't hold 1.48. I didn't get off. Never get off. If someone whacks you, never stay down. I think my friend Micky Burton – we stood together at the Battle of Ballymore, Brisbane, in 1975, during which match he became the first England player ever to get sent off – wrote a book with that title. He also wrote me a kind letter, and it was in joined-up writing and everything.

I dropped the pace to 1 min. 59 sec. I just couldn't, just couldn't. Please. Please. Go slower than 2 min. at this level of effort. The metres ticked by, I felt a bit better. Here I am, the walking pharmacy, full of poison to apoptosise the rogue cells wherever they may be in my body. God, let there be no sharks in Kalamata Bay. The metres roll off, the end is in sight and I squeeze the pace down to 1 min. 50 sec. Should I be doing this? 11 min. 16 sec. – that's an average of about 1 min. 52.5 sec. per 500 m. I took my pulse, fingers on the throat, count for 15 seconds, wait for 45, then count again. One minute – 164 pulse. Two minutes – 124 pulse. Three minutes – 106 pulse. Four minutes – 88 pulse. Such a slow recovery. You can gauge your fitness by the recovery of your heart rate. I am in a different world from where I used to be, which I'd better get used to. I'd agreed with the bouncy prof to stay on the poison for three years, and if I get IMRT'd in January, this will come with its own bag of side effects. Hey, I'll take it all and more if it means I can live.

Most people's average pulse is 72 beats per minute. Many people who, like me, train hard would take pride in the fact that their average resting pulse rate is about half this figure. When you're exercising, a crude measure is to take your age away from 220, so in my case that's 163. This is your maximum heart rate. To get the best in training, you should put in steady effort at about 80 per cent of your max heart rate; this for me would be about 130 beats per minute. I know all this, but have always gone for just a few beats below my maximum. Maybe that's why I'm now picking up the tab. After 20 years of contact sport, my knees are shot to bits. Would it have been better not to have fallen in love with sport, any sport? Nah! Wouldn't have missed it for all the world. But where do you draw the line between sporting excellence and self-harm?

After the erg session I go to meet Paul, who has spent more time than most considering that question. It's a warm day, but he's in a suit and a mac, carrying a big bag. I was already smiling but now I am beginning to grin. He's flown in from Dublin, where he lives surrounded by his close extended family. He's a feature writer for the *Sunday Times* and I'm a station on his line, his next trick. I'm flattered; he's hit some pretty impressive stations. Without being too Uriah Heepish, why me, Lord? I played rugby about 30 years ago for England, had my 15 minutes on *Superstars* and have done a bit of puffing on some commercial gym kit. Not exactly David Beckham. Got cancer, but cancer isn't that exclusive – there are lots of us in the Club.

Then again, I don't care why I'm now walking down Jermyn Street with Paul because this 43-year-old man in a mac who doesn't know where Eros is – doesn't know it! – has, since about 1990, been my hero. Maybe.

We stumble into the back entrance of Fortnum & Mason's, amongst the old, genteel, mainly female clientele, and sit at a corner table. I don't tell him he's my hero, maybe. Instead I tell him what he'll order for lunch. There are seven starters, seven mains. I guess he'll order salmon fishcakes and Dover sole off the bone. I get it right. I am feeling so clever; I've never, ever got it right before. Today, I did.

In 1990, Paul Kimmage wrote a book called *Rough Ride*, and in 2001, Martin Cross wrote a book called *Olympic Obsession*. There is nothing wrong with sporting heroes writing or having ghosted Christmas stocking fillers, and some are very good. There is a market, and there are products. Fine. But these two books (and there are probably other examples) bleed. The personal cost involved in writing them must have been huge. Paul thinks he's going to interview me for the *Sunday Times*. Wrong. They're just picking up the tab for the fishcakes and Dover sole. I'm interviewing Paul, 'cause I want to find out about him, I want to know stuff. I want to get rid of 'maybe'.

We natter. At three o'clock he says, you know, the interview hasn't started. Oh yes it has, Paul. He takes out his pad and tape machine and does his job, which he is good at. You don't stay features writer of a leading paper for long if you aren't good at what you do.

Five o'clock. The genteel ladies taking tea, who remind me of my mum, may or may not notice the animated pair in the corner. I've got a meeting of Tideway Scullers president's committee in Wardour Street at 7.30, so we leave the corner table and drift into Soho and sit and have an espresso at a table outside a café. We say goodbye at about 7.15. We've both enjoyed the day.

Paul was born in Dublin on 7 May 1962 with bike riding in his genes. Throughout his life, his father told him, 'In cycling there is more heartbreak than happiness.'

I may very well be a member of East Grinstead Cycling Club, who used to ride in their 10-mile Tuesday-evening summer pursuits and got John Hutt, who owned Allin's Cycles in Croydon (and who died of cancer about 10 years ago) to build me a 27.5-in.-frame Allin 735, but I don't know too much about cycling. However, I can recognise a gypsy dog – all ribs and cock – when I see one.

At 19, Paul was Irish amateur cycling champion. If you want to read all the details of his cycling read his book – but it's not about the book. Riding professionally for the RMO team in the 1986 Tour de France, Paul finished 131st out of 132 riders. Three years later, on 13 July during Stage 12, Toulouse to Montpellier, he steps off his bike ashamed and broken-hearted. His dad was right: heartbreak.

But why was his heart broken? Because he wasn't good enough? Because a gypsy dog doesn't have a pedigree? Because he got off the machine, when you never stay down? Well, maybe and maybe and maybe. In life, we all sometimes get to win, and that is easy and should be enjoyed, particularly as much of life is learning to deal with losing. But the real mark of a person is not how they deal with winning or losing, it's how they deal with injustice. In this case, the injustice of having to compete on a skewed playing field.

Am I heading here towards Henry Newbolt territory – 'Play up, play up and play the game'? I don't think so. Paul Kimmage did not play up, play up and play the game. He did the exact opposite. He not only spat in the soup, he gobbed in the faces of the professional cycling world, with his book *Rough Ride*, written in 1990. I read the book when it was first published and loved it. Kimmage was one of the first insiders to break the cycling world's silence on the subject of drugs.

I wanted to find out why he wrote it. Was it just a stepping stone to a literary career? Was it for personal gain, because actually he wasn't good enough or strong enough or talented enough to stay on his bike? Was he hurting people who want heroes, however flawed? And because of my glorious cancer, I was able to sit with him in Fortnum & Mason's department store and find out about 'maybe'.

Brilliant news: there is no maybe. It's unequivocal. Paul Kimmage is a hero.

There is a case to be made for saying, why not take performance-enhancing drugs? Why not go faster, higher, quicker with a bit of help from your friends?

Why not turn sport into part of the entertainment freak show? People have always had a morbid curiosity to see the bearded lady or Christians being eaten by lions. So why not?

The reason is simple. I'm now a walking chemist's shop. The poison I'm taking is keeping me alive at a price. I have to pay that price; it extends the string. Young men and women shouldn't have to pay that price.

If doping becomes the norm then everyone is in the circus and all of us will suffer for it, and none more so than the – albeit willingly exploited – marionettes. We are all diminished. Maybe the top of the marionettes' ladder isn't for the moment too unhappy with the way things are, but what about the B team, the guys who have to join in with the rules of the show just to stay in it, even when where they are is effectively nowhere? And what is the price they'll pay?

In cycling alone, Johannes Draaijer, Bert Oosterbosch and Joachim Halupczok all went to bed and never woke up. And there is a long list of other B-team professionals, young men you'll never have heard of, who died as a result of performance-enhancing drugs. Human growth hormone is not your friend; neither is the other testosterone-based oxygen-enhancer EPO your friend.

At play, EPO allows oxygen into the blood; at rest, it turns the blood to treacle. Slow heart rates go even slower, the body cannot work to counteract blood clots. Into the heart, through the lungs to pick up oxygen, and then the clots hit the lung capillaries and block them. If they are lucky, these young men don't wake up, but probably they do, with huge pains in their chest, fighting for breath in a hotel room, a fight they lose. Tell me, does a young kid with dreams and hopes, but who is in reality just making up the numbers, deserve that?

The guys who take or have taken EPO to go quicker, faster, higher – who is going to care when they suffer from a whole series of unpleasant conditions in later life? Who is going to pick up the bill? No one but them. No one, as the spotlight moves on and each generation finds its own sporting heroes. Performance-enhancing drugs are poison with baggage. They can kill, but they also have effects that will only be felt when no one cares and no one sees, or even bothers to look.

Wednesday, 12 October 2005

05.35. I wake up before the alarm goes and look at the accusing orange figures glowing in the dark. The light early mornings have been lost some time ago, and so the figures now glow. But I've got the drop on those orange figures: it isn't 05.35, it is actually 05.30. Why are these five minutes so cosy? Why are they so precious? To us, that is, who play this game of horological delusion. Last night, for the first time in a long time, I didn't get up to go to the toilet. Then again, I went to bed at quarter past midnight.

I creep out of cosy land, pick up some clothes from the landing, where I put them last night (well, early this morning, actually) and gently edge down the stairs in the dark, feeling my way with my feet. Is it like this for Eric every moment of every day?

Into the kitchen, light on, kettle on, toaster, three slices. One slice of toast for Torben, who now has a pink collar. He's been castrated, too, but physically and not chemically. I notice for the first time his dick has shrunk. He hasn't even got a towel to cover his shame. Blimey! Looking at a dog's genitals at 5.40 in the morning must be the first step on the road to somewhere unpleasant.

I take the car, too tired for the bike. It's just getting light as I arrive at Tideway Scullers at 6.45. Rak is there early; apart from our age and a willingness to turn up, maybe we don't have so much in common, but we've been rowing together happily now for about ten years. Rak is a lawyer. One of Ian Robertson's usual opening space fillers (for example, at the Lions lunch) can and often is adapted to be about lawyers. Ian was making the fairly unoriginal point that chartered accountants are pretty dull and tedious. However, he suggested, although accountants may be dull, they are not as bad as lawyers, who are complete tossers. Ian told us, the assembled diners, that when he had made this point during another speech, a man who seemed to be upset had approached him afterwards and said, 'I take great exception to that statement,' to which Ian said, 'I suppose you're a lawyer.' The offended man replied, 'No, I am not a lawyer. I, sir, am a complete tosser.' Yeah, well, I suppose you had to be there. Strange that it's now illegal to tell jokes about religion but you can mock lawyers or accountants all you like – that is, until this government brings in some legislation criminalising jokes about people's employment.

Rak calls the shots, and it's a pyramid down to Hammersmith against the strong flow and a steady row back down the middle of the river at about 27, over the same course we followed on Saturday. I feel surprisingly good. All things considered.

Rak likes films and stories and rowing. He has four children and is part of a close family. For some reason, as we put the boat back in the shed, he tells me a story based around a text from the Koran (Somerset Maugham wrote a version of it, a story called 'The Appointment in Samarra'). Two men, a master and his servant, were riding towards Mecca when they met Death, who had a surprised expression on his face. The master turned his horse away from Death and raced away to Samarra. The servant looked at Death and said, 'Why were you so startled to see my master?' Death said, 'I was surprised to see him here on the road to Mecca, as I have an appointment with him tonight in Samarra.'

For some reason, I seem to attract tales of mortality. I'm like that character in the Monty Python sketch, Arthur 'Two Sheds' Jackson, the joke being based around the fact that no matter what the subject, the conversation always comes back round to his two sheds.

Am I Andy 'Mortality' Ripley?

It's eight o'clock. Quick shower – no one around, praise the Lord – and into the Hogarth Road traffic jam. I'm on my way to Westbourne Studios in Notting Hill to meet Will, who got married on 4 June and was still dancing when I was being morphined, oxygened and heparined up in East Surrey Hospital in the early hours of 5 June. Will, Julian and Alex sit on the board of Sharpcards.com with Loz (but she's in New York) and me. The three of them have a lot in common. They are all about 30, have all recently got married and have babies, are all, against the odds, having passed on sensible careers – lawyer, banker and chartered accountant – trying to start things up that belong largely to themselves. They have all to date had lucky and fortunate lives and educations. It is a little bit like the set of *Friends*.

Alex is married to Amelia, who is one of my sister Eileen's four daughters. Which is indirectly how I come to be in the daily traffic jam on the A4, now just past the Hogarth Roundabout. I am hugely flattered that all of them have asked me to be involved in their dreams. I genuinely don't know why they've done it, but I love it. They even give me a few quid; I'd pay to be there.

Will started Sharpcards about five years ago in the dot-com boom days. It was an Internet site for people who were too lazy to go to the shops to buy greetings cards. You would log onto the site, see a huge range of cards, select one, say what you wanted written in it and where you wanted it sent, pay via PayPal – about £2 – and Sharpos would do the rest. Which they did.

Half a million quid to build the site and back-up delivery system and about £20,000 a month in gross running costs means you have to sell about 300 cards a day, every day, day after day, to break even. As with most start-ups, the question is, can you build up sales so you cover costs before you run out of cash? Sharpcards, unlike most dot-com companies, actually did break even in February and December, thanks to Christmas cards and St Valentine's Day, but two months out of twelve doesn't lead to spreadsheet-projection heaven. Loads of Internet-based companies, a couple of which I'd been only too familiar with, had had to roll over, with all the associated acrimony and gnashing of teeth. Will got lucky. Having survived in this environment, established a name and experience in greetings cards, he approached mobile-phone operators. They'd deal with Will, Loz, Julian and Alex because they had earned a reputation, had first-hand knowledge of Internet and mobile markets and technology and were fun. Essentially, operators own a stretch of road on which they want to see traffic – games, ringtones, wallpaper and greetings – and the revenue that flows from that traffic. Will got a number of yearly contracts to supply greetings traffic to some of the operators.

I believe one reason mobile-phone users use downloaded greetings, which can cost up to £3 a go, is as follows (incidentally, if you are a prostate-cancer sufferer and over 60, or even if you are neither and all this is of mind-boggling dullness, skip a page or two – I honestly don't mind): it's flirting. If you meet someone you take a shine to, if you ask them out directly, face to face, eye to eye, however euphemistically you put it, asking, for example, 'Would you like to go out for a drink?', they may just say no. Rejected. Crushed or what? Much easier on all parties if you wimp out and send a text message. Which many do. Even better, if you know they are, say, a Millwall fan, download an image of a Millwall shirt, add a message, perhaps saying, 'Saw this and it reminded me of you.' Well, no rejection – you've opened up a dialogue and shown you are willing to make an investment.

Obviously, not everyone is a Millwall supporter, but all Sharpcards has to do is provide whatever it is the market wants and make sure the goods are put in a place where users will see them. Now everybody is happy. The user has made contact and not risked losing face through rejection. The operator gets half the download charge and increases traffic on the string, as the recipient can use the greeting as often as they like at no further charge to them. Sharpcards has a revenue stream, as long as it keeps providing state-of-the-art greetings, and now does make enough in revenue to cover its costs and to fund an office in the US to do the same over there. Might work.

So I get to Westbourne Studios, with its twenty or so businesses, at nine and meet Julian in the lift. He is on his way to Cardiff. His company is Red Snappers, for whom my daughters were taking pictures at the Oval.

I sit down in the communal café area with Will and Alex. I must be about 25 years older than anybody else in the large, odd-shaped room. It reminds me of being in the café at the Judge Institute, the business school at Cambridge, surrounded by youthful excitement. I really like it.

They ask me how I am. My usual reply now is, on the hormone treatment, seems to be going well, if it works out I'll have some radiotherapy treatment after Christmas, and, who knows, I could get away with this. I never say that there may be sharks in Kalamata Bay. With these guys, though, I like to play. I tell them at length how if I didn't have cancer, I wouldn't have gone to the NHS interview or be about to go to Cadiz or have met Paul Kimmage in Fortnum & Mason's for lunch yesterday or received such kindnesses or felt so alive as I do now. Will says, yeah, well, maybe it's not that other people are nicer, maybe you're nicer, and, hey, that wouldn't be difficult; people are just reacting to your new niceness. We have a board meeting.

I drive home, tired.

If I'm tired, I just go and rest for a while – seems sensible. It's what anyone does if they're tired.

Early afternoon, looking out of the window onto the garden. I live and have lived for the last 25 years in the front bit of Morven House. The back has been divided into two separate homes and the stables and gatehouse are also separate properties, but we have the front bit. There is a sweeping gravelled drive, the house is three storeys high and white and Georgian, and visitors think we are really rich. Which in some ways we are. Step a bit closer, and you see the house is one room deep and rather like a Wild West cowboy-film street set – all front and no substance. We love it, and the front garden was planted when the house was built in about 1832. There is a massive copper beech, a cedar, an enormous Wellingtonia (said by Andy Gale, from whom we bought the house, to be the tallest tree in Surrey) and a mass of rhododendrons and azaleas. It is wonderful at any time of the year but especially now as the Japanese maple turns to red and the birches shuffle their turning coats. So I just look out and count my blessings and thank Ho Chee.

Ho Chee was born in Canton (now Guangzhou) in 1789. He became friendly with John Elphinstone, son of a director of the East India Company, and himself a supercargo with the company in Canton. John Elphinstone, who was an earnest evangelical Christian, retired from the East India Company due to ill health in 1818. In 1819, aged 30, Ho Chee, who had converted to the Christian faith, joined Elphinstone in England. Perhaps surprisingly, as at this time there was little love lost between the British and the Chinese, Ho Chee stayed in England and married in 1823. He and his wife had eight children and lived in Nortons (Morven House). Periodically, descendants of Ho Chee knock on the door. We have collected a small file of notes and letters and photos which we will leave to the next people to enjoy Ho Chee's legacy and wonderful trees.

But right now, at this moment in time, looking out of the window, I am the beneficiary of that legacy.

Thursday, 13 October 2005

The best sort of day: empty and stretching out to be filled. I have learned to build a whole day around going to buy a postage stamp and feeling a huge sense of achievement when I complete this demanding task, which can somehow take days to get done. A job well done. As Elizabeth Smart wrote, although not about buying a stamp:

> That day I finished
> A small piece
> For an obscure magazine
> I popped it in the box
>
> And such a starry elation
> Came over me . . .
> . . .
> That the freedom and force it engendered
> Shone and spun
> Out of my old raincoat.
>
> It must have looked like love
> Or a fabulous free holiday
> To the young men sauntering
> Down Berwick Street.
> . . .
> But done done done
> Everything in the world
> Flowed back
> Like a huge bonus.

Good old Canadian Elizabeth, fell in love with a married poet, followed her heart, wrote *By Grand Central Station I Sat Down and Wept*, had four children, then lived in Suffolk in a house in a dell with no road to it and tended her garden till she died. Voltaire would have been proud.

I can do proud. The erg two days ago still rankled, so

I decided to do a steady 2,000 m at around 1 min. 48 sec. per 500 m – that's 7 min. 12 sec. from start to completion. Before 4 June, I would have done a steady 2,000 m at around 1 min. 40 sec. per 500 m – that's 6 min. 40 sec. from start to completion. Really going for it, I would have hoped to do about 1 min. 35 sec. per 500m – that's 6 min. 20 sec.

Now, all these numbers may be mind-bogglingly tedious and meaningless unless you happen to be a fellow erg geek. However, what they do tell me is that my loss in physical ability is probably due not to the cancer – it would have set in before 4 June if that had been the case – but to the effects of warfarin and Zoladex.

I did the 2,000 m and didn't feel too bad, and in a time of 7 min. 7.5 sec. That's about 27.5 sec. slower than I would have taken if I'd never bust my ribs, had a pulmonary embolism or been stuck on hormone therapy. Allowing, say, 6 sec. for the lack of training and one or two for the ageing process, that means I have lost about 20 sec. in total or 5 sec. per 500 m due to the side effects of the drugs that are keeping me in with a shout of staying alive. So that's a loss of between 3 and 4 per cent directly attributable to the drugs.

The question is, of course, will it be 4 per cent every four months or is that it – a loss of 4 per cent and now I'm just on a lower plateau? Let's take the plateau theory as the given: so now I should readjust all my training schedules to take account of a 4 per cent drug-deficit margin. This is huge. My time last year at the UK national championships was 6 min. 23 sec.; flat out, trained and hurting, adding in my drug margin, for the same effort it would now be 6 min. 38 sec.

I wonder if the benefits of taking testosterone/EPO give a similar positive uplift. Last year, at a time of 6 min. 23 sec., if I had taken EPO, would my time have been 3 to 4 per cent better, that's to say 6 min. 10 sec.? Clearly, the potential drug enhancement would be less predictable than I'm assuming for the purposes of argument here, but, hey, we are in theory land. It's just a common-or-garden hypothesis, based neither on fact or even anecdotal evidence. Still . . . Imagine you are a massively talented young male 100-m sprinter who trains his nuts off and has a personal best of, say, 10.02 sec. Someone says, 'Take this, this is just a sweet,' and you improve your time by 0.97 per cent to 9.76 sec. From world-class international athlete to intergalactic superstar. The world wants intergalactic superstars.

However, the reality is more likely to be that you are a good athlete with dreams and a PB of 10.4 sec., you eat the sweet and do 10.1 – still just making up the numbers. You're tossed away when you're used up, and if you get really unlucky, one night, aged 25, you go to bed and don't wake up.

Saturday, 15 October 2005

Winnie Churchill said, 'Success is the ability to go from one failure to another with no loss of enthusiasm.' By his definition, I've had a pretty successful day: stumbling through a couple of failures without any loss of enthusiasm, ending up with a shining reason why I've always loved sport and then finally a bit of shameful self-discovery.

First failure: I got the letter from the NHS Appointments Commission. Binned. A 'Dear John'. Not good enough. Well, rejection is always a bitter pill, but the less vain, more practical part of me did heave a small sigh of relief. I had made the effort to help as a thank you (and I still feel a huge indebtedness to the NHS), but there was obviously a better candidate, and I sincerely wish the successful applicant good luck.

Being a non-exec in an NHS trust is a labour of love. Who in their right minds would want to be in that firing line over the next five years? Thank goodness, however, that there are people who are prepared to stand up and be counted. Bless them.

Second failure: I had been on the Railtrack Private Shareholders Action Group (RPSAG) for the last five years or so. The group had been set up in the wake of Railtrack's collapse following the withdrawal of government support in 2001. The ordinary shareholders felt that the Government had forced Railtrack into administration without any intention of properly compensating shareholders. We were referred to by one adviser to the Treasury as 'the grannies who will lose their blouses'. There were actually 250,000 of us grannies and we got organised. Some 55,000 of us whacked in 10p a share, giving us a fund of £2 million, and set up RPSAG. We were threatened with massive legal costs, but we, the grannies, put a minister (Transport Secretary Stephen Byers) in the dock to account for his actions, the first time this had ever been done in Britain. Today, however, Justice Lindsay's report was made public, and the judge has dismissed RPSAG's claim.

So, two failures. But now for the sport. The sun's beam is dancing on the sparkling Thames at Chiswick as Stefanos and I look down from the balcony outside Tideway Scullers. The river is alive with boats waiting for the 2.30 start of the Pairs Head. It is more a summer's day than a summer's day, warm and gentle and bright, with a soft wind blowing over the quickly ebbing tide, ruffling up the water. Rak and I are number 330 in a race of 340 boats – women and children first and old men (veterans aged 55–60) at the back. With 15 seconds between each boat, we won't start until about 3.45, so we'll wait and then boat at about 3.30, hopefully without the marshal noticing.

Stefanos is 37, Greek, charming, bright, big, has a PhD in something or other and is with his son Nicholas, who is 9. Stefanos seems to have a number of wives, but, hey, who's counting, and I'm sure everyone is very happy. We usually row together as part of a coxless four, but today Stefanos isn't competing. A month ago, he was at the world veteran championships in Glasgow, where someone in a pub whacked him over the head with a bottle from behind. Hello, Stefanos, welcome to Glasgow. So he is watching with his son and getting better. Stefanos has been in the Greek navy, so I ask him on the balcony if there are sharks in Greece. Yes, of course. My right shoulder felt cold.

Number 330. Go. Two long draw strokes, nothing fancy, hands away, quickly round the turn, square early, slowly down the slide, drop it in short, leave it out there, arms loose and straight, connect with the back, drive with the legs, feel the water moving underneath the boat, quick hands, slowly lengthen out, it's 4 km to Hammersmith Bridge, keep the rate up but not too high. Smooth, hands away, body over, down the slide, square, remember to breathe, squeeze away from 331, squeeze away from 331. Closing on both 329 and 328, approaching Barnes Bridge middle arch, steering, that's Rak's problem, I'll just row. Steady head, keep the rate up, water now really beginning to lump up, sweat dripping into my eyes. I love it, I am alive. Breathing hard, quick hands, past the bandstand, pulling away from 328 and 329, who are two lengths astern, closing on 324 at the changeover. Wait to take the rate up half a pip at the end of the Eyot, don't rush it, wait for it, 324 not giving up or giving way, don't break the rhythm. End of the Eyot, next stroke, legs on. Pull away from 324, on 327's stern, opposite St Paul's School's hard. Two minutes to the bridge, don't go early, wait, breathe in, now like James Brown take it to the bridge, take it to the bridge, quick hands, be strong, lengthen out, empty the tank, leave 327. Light.

Showered, cleaned up, sitting in the clubhouse, feeling good, mellow, results available tomorrow on the Net. Bothered? Not really. Just good to be there. This is where I want to be; this is who I now am.

At home in the dying hours of the busy day. Over the last few days, Gloria Hunniford has been puffing her new book about her daughter Caron Keating dying of cancer. She knows how to puff: radio, newspapers and TV. Right now, she's on Parkinson. I'm about to zap, 'cause for some reason I don't like it. Is she someone using her grief to make a few bob, chasing the fading spotlight? I don't zap.

I couldn't have been more wrong. It takes a nanosecond to see that this is a woman in pain. This is all and the best she can do to remember her beloved daughter. I feel ashamed of myself for being so cynical. My heart goes out to a mother who has lost both a beloved daughter and the sparkle in her now sad eyes. It is so hard for all those whose loved ones have this disease, but a parent grieving over a child . . . I switch off and pray for Gloria and all sufferers.

Sunday, 16 October 2005

Something is happening here. When I started this record, it was essentially that: a recording of dates and what drugs I was taking and what was happening to me, so I could better understand and perhaps even rationalise or at least try to come to terms with change and the changes that were happening to me and the changes that might happen to me.

Now I seem to be writing down, recording, every moment of my life and the people in that moment and how I arrived at that moment in time. Is this not a burden, a self-inflicted albatross, a self-diminishing therapeutic obsession?

Has life become so precious that every moment is precious? Am I so fearful that I don't want an instant to be lost? Am I so frightened that this is my only way of dealing with it? Am I scared that I will be forgotten? We are all eventually going to be forgotten. Who knows where their great-grandfather is buried?

I had resolved to miss a day or two out and live in the land of throwaway fact and forgotten action and not just in a hard-drive-stored, cloistered record. But this evening, when Clouds had gone back to Bath and Stef was sitting on the sofa (another one) in my metaphoric shed, she said, 'Are you going to write about today?' I said no; she said, 'Oh, go on, Dad.' So, my beloved Stef, this is just for you.

We went to church together. I was in a crazy rush because I was doing the second reading and didn't know what it was and you said, Stef, as I was rushing, 'Can I come too?' Well, no one goes to church with me. You kids just don't, and Elisabeth, even though she believes in stuff, she doesn't like the hymns or the peace. But Elisabeth, like the shepherds, just doesn't question anything, she just is a Christian. Me, I'm like the wise men (obviously); I'm taking ages to get there, following that star.

We get to the church. It is so warm and sunny. I practise my piece. It's St Paul's first letter to the Thessalonians, Chapter 1, Verses 1 to 10. Hope and discipline. In my frame of mind I'll clutch at any straw.

After the service, before we go to visit Mum's grave (though we actually know she's not there, she is at the Wash Pool on Cleeve Hill in the Cotswolds), I am so proud of you, talking and being and smiling; you are now a woman. Then afterwards, sitting in the car which took the sofa to Austria, good car, you share with me your hopes of getting a good degree at UEA to add to your record of never getting less than an A in school exams and how you would like to do a doctorate and be Dr Stefanie Ripley by the time you are 24. My heart is breaking because I, like your mum, don't care what you become, I just love you as you are, and I want to be there always, forever, to pick you up when you fall down. As you will, as we all do. So who will be there to pick you up, Stef? I suppose, like all of us, you have to learn to pick yourself up, and you will.

At lunch, outside, it's warm – all of us and Mouse's girlfriend, Bryony. Mouse is still going on about 'What is a monger?' There's a fishmonger (trout for lunch), an ironmonger, a warmonger and, Mum added in, a scaremonger; but he doesn't know what a monger is. He is getting very boring, as in, 'Could you monger me the potatoes?' You, Stef, then ask Bryony the name of her cousin in Norwich. 'It's Hattie.' You are seized with a fit of the giggles and say, 'What's her brother called, Scarfie?'

We walk over the hills just before dusk and the rain, over the field where the new farmer has ploughed up the footpaths, past Jen's place, round the hill and through the wood. Torben loves it, so do we and as always we talk about stuff. You then tell me about your friend Claire's stepdad who had prostate cancer, a few years ago. PSA 57, radical prostatectomy, didn't work, followed by hormone treatment. He then died. I know eventually you'll be able to handle anything.

The other thing that happened yesterday was that Clouds said she was going to enter for the British Indoor Rowing Championships in mid-November. Two years of good intentions, but actually of drinking and clubbing, haven't got her in the best shape. She started on Saturday and today did a 19-minute pyramid session. The machine was lying about, and I asked Mouse to do a 500-m piece; he said OK. Almost without trying, he pulled 1 min. 19 sec. Unbelievable.

Monday, 17 October 2005

Yesterday, I resolved to stop writing about each day and to live my life for a while. But first of all, I will get on the Net to find out about sharks in Kalamata Bay, and then I will think about God and death and find the answer to that one by, say, dinner. Then I'll think about me and how others see me. Tomorrow, I'm going to drive to Cornwall and stop off to see some friends, then meet up with my brother and sisters for a few days. After that, going to Cadiz to sail the 800 miles to Las Palmas with a man I've met for 20 minutes. I'll see how Jonathan and the crew are with me and maybe write about it later or maybe just stop writing this diary and live. First, two loose ends: sharks and God.

Well, I suppose we are all scared of the future, uncertainty, the dark, what we don't understand. Perhaps scared is the wrong word, maybe it's apprehensive, maybe it's something else altogether. Old people like me are concerned, maybe that's the word, about being alone, having no money, ill health; these are not the troubles of youth, when you worry about things like sharks or not jumping through academic hoops or your friends not liking you, or your mum letting you down. Different stuff, but it's the same – uncertainty.

Rational thought is a crumbling crutch against the imagined strength of a particular and specific uncertainty and whether that specific uncertainty is real or just imaginary, in your head there is no difference. It's just scary.

So my right shoulder hurts. I know I have locally advanced prostate cancer, but has it now metastasised into my shoulder? Have I moved a step nearer the exit?

I believed there were no sharks in Kalamata Bay. Well, if you go onto the Net and feed in 'shark attacks Mediterranean', you'll find that after a short while your attitude towards sharks and my contrived metaphor fades fast. There are in fact many species of sharks, including great white sharks (*Carcharodon carcharias*) in that sea.

On the other hand, according to one site, between 1890 and 2003 there were only five reported incidents involving sharks around the whole of Greece, the most recent being over 25 years ago, in the summer of 1981, a non-fatal nip at Pagasitikos Kolpos, near Volos. In truth, it is the plight of sharks in the Mediterranean, and other marine creatures – be they loggerhead turtles, monk seals or striped dolphins – that should really be of concern to my daughter Stef. Still, we can't be certain of anything. Will the dawn break tomorrow?

Another thought occurs to me about Stef. When we go back to Seefeld in winter, most days Stef goes out skiing or snowboarding. She only has to look in Mouse's room to see all the plaster casts he has saved from his snowboarding and mountain biking injuries, to see how dangerous it is. The statistics for injury or death caused by winter sports are usually given as 1 per 1.5 million ski excursions. Well, if a ski season is from December to March that's 120 days, and if Seefeld has 10,000 ski guests, then in that village alone, statistically, there will be one death from skiing almost every year, never mind the mass of knee (skiers) and wrist (boarders) injuries. Is Stef scared? Not a bit. It's the dark, it's the unknown, it's uncertainty that's scary.

Although there is no certainty, we have to behave as if dawn will come tomorrow, we have to assume there are no sharks in Kalamata Bay, and I have to assume that the pain in my shoulder is just a pain in my shoulder. Otherwise, we will sink into a morass of unjustified doubts and darkness and what life we have left will just pass us by, spent in a state of anxiety.

So, God and death before dinner. It would be presumptuous of me to imagine that just because my mortality is in question I have any great insight. I mean, if I was a nit before now, with a few ill-founded, pretentious ideas, maybe I am now not an insightful nit but merely a potentially dying nit. Although I believe it was Samuel Johnson who said that a man who is to be hanged in the morning has a focused mind. I feel focused.

People down the ages have always tried to resolve the question of uncertainty. So rites, ritual, religion, astrology have all given comfort. Birth and death have been the major events, with all that stuff in between called life. Birth – miraculous and difficult as it is – is less contentious, because if you're reading this, it has already happened; that just leaves the uncertainty of death and the time between now and then.

So death is the big one. The great buildings of the world, from the pyramids to the Taj Mahal, speak of our fear of and preoccupation with death. Lucky charms, astrology and most of the other comfort-givers step away from this question, leaving, out on its own ahead of the game, religion.

The question that people, because of all animals we alone have free will and the ability to reason, must have asked, across cultures and languages, and which has come cascading down through time must be 'Is this it?' Is there some point to all of this? To life? Religion has played a key role in this questioning because it has addressed the problem, has told us unequivocally (great word) that beyond death there is life in some shape or other. This, over time, has proven to be a winning marketing strategy.

All the great religions of the world offer hope of some kind of afterlife, and all have their different requirements for entry. For Christians, baptism is the route. If you are baptised and live your life according to the Bible, particularly following its teaching that you should love the Lord your God with all your heart and your neighbour as yourself, then, if you have faith, you are promised eternal salvation.

To some, the primary requirement of religion is that you must first suspend rational belief. Hegel and later Marx saw religion merely as a method by which the ruling elites subjugated the masses, who would put up with anything in this life and, crucially, behave in a way that would preserve the status quo in order to gain entry into the life to come. Atheism was one of the cornerstones of communist doctrine. Atheists are simply people who have no need for a belief in God. It's brave to be an atheist. An agnostic, meanwhile, is one who believes that it is impossible to know whether there is a God. Atheists are not people who are angry at God for something; that is apostasy.

God is not an objective fact that is supported by overwhelming evidence. Atheists would suggest faith in God helps believers to make sense of the world. To believers, the statement 'I believe in God' is a statement about ourselves, not about God. An atheist might suggest that the religious find it useful to believe there is some sort of higher force that brings some sort of order to their lives that they cannot find on their own. Maybe they're right – it's ultimately a question of faith; but I know I have far more in common with a Jew or Muslim than an atheist.

What kind of Christian am I? Well, not a very good

one. My mum took us to the local church in Liverpool (St Peter's, Woolton) and then Bristol (St Alban's). At the onset of puberty, I found better things to do.

My mum and dad were both born in the Edwardian period. It was la belle époque, but there probably wasn't too much belle époquing going on in their lives. But that period, before the First World War, must have seen Europe in general and Britain in particular at its political, industrial and cultural zenith. Wealth trickling down from the trade and exploitation of other countries and other classes, technology leaping ahead with all sorts of goodies. A rigid class system so everyone knew their place, rampant nationalism, a sense of duty and order, and a religious hierarchy defended, supported and unthreatened by the state. The nineteenth century had belonged to the Western European nations as, after the First World War, the twentieth was to belong to the United States and in due course, I imagine, the twenty-first will to Asia.

The late Victorians and Edwardians had seen a great questioning of religion and ideas about the afterlife, and they certainly posed that question 'Is this it?' At the same time, there was a great increase in church building and society was overwhelmingly religious, and my parents and grandparents must have been swept up in that culture. They went to church and therefore so did I, until puberty.

My mum found great comfort in the church all her life, I think more as a social outlet than a religious experience; she loved the community of the church. Was she a Christian with agnostic tendencies or an agnostic with Christian leanings? I don't know. I'll have to ask her when I see her next.

Dinner is ready and I'll leave these questions for you to answer. I do know I want to be buried in the local churchyard at St John's, Dormansland. But not yet.

Monday, 7 November 2005

I felt I was wandering, so I haven't written anything for three weeks, and now I'm in my room, looking out of the window, early winter, weak sun in the late afternoon (actually, it's only 3.30, but with the nights drawing in and the clocks going back, it feels later). I'll make a wood fire. It's just me and Elisabeth and Torben in Ho Chee's house. Elisabeth has bought some mussels from the fish man, and there's a bottle of cold white wine in the fridge. Cosy. I feel strong, four months to the day since my first shot of Zoladex.

And, like the moth to the candle, I have been drawn back to this record of mine. I don't know whether it's yet another side effect of the hormone treatment, but I'm feeling very sensitive, almost bright. I know I am becoming self-obsessed and living in a private world, in my head, but I like it. I can be all those things I was always too frightened to be – pretentious, opinionated, prejudiced. It's such a freedom, such a release not having to bother when you step on someone's toes, not having to pretend to care. This next bit is even more about me. I've shamelessly used the last three weeks to find the answer to the question 'Who am I?' Peer Gynt eat your heart out.

Monday, 17 October 2005

(but written on 7 November 2005)

For me, friends and music are people you met and records you heard before you were 30. After that, it's really just good acquaintances and good sounds.

Is it something to do with a shared history? Is it something to do with an age when you were more vulnerable? Maybe less world-weary, more open, more available? They knew you before, in that other country called youth and dreams. If I met most of my friends now, we would probably pass like cars in the day on the M25. Those old friends almost become like family, even better maybe, as there is no sense of duty or obligation, as there is or at least should be in a family.

So Elisabeth and I drive down to the New Forest to see George Lloyd-Roberts for lunch. I always felt I had let George down one evening about 1975 at the Brewery Field in Bridgend.

He was a gym-built tight-head prop with a very powerful upper body. He was also kinda lippy, genuinely double-barrelled, a Lloyd's insurance underwriter in the City and just the sort of target any self-respecting Welsh front row would want to give a right good seeing to. Particularly as he was English (well, actually he's from North Wales, but whatever, he obviously needed, and periodically needs, a good shoeing).

Now, being lippy can take many different forms, but I think the most offensive is as follows. So this match, just outside Bridgend, just outside Swansea, just outside the fast lane of life. The first scrum of the wet evening match, in our 22, our put-in, home referee, no cameras, no independent linesmen (it's a friendly). Lionel Weston, our scrum-half, puts the ball into the scrum. Phil Keith-Roach, our hooker – this was in the days of the hooking front row rather than the shoving front row – heels it back.

Their second row has slipped his binding and is giving Phil an introduction to the next 80 minutes at the Brewery Field, but he misses and hits George, quite hard. George then says, in his expensive and beautifully pronounced English, and this is lippy beyond lippydom, he says, 'I say, was that really necessary?'

The Welsh eight erupted with a might born of 500 years of English exploitation and oppression, all of which rage fell on George. Owen Glendower would have been well pleased.

Here is the guilty bit: the other seven of us forwards, instead of standing by our man like Tammy Wynette, took the ball and, as there were now fourteen of us and only seven of them, their eight forwards being occupied giving George a well-deserved kicking, we managed to score in the far corner. The brave fourteen, walking back in triumph, noticed a large battered, bloodied lump at the top left-hand side of the field, which said in its beautifully pronounced English, 'Well done.' A.K. Rodgers, who had a degree in English from Ealing Poly, suggested that this was an example of irony and we all ought to give George another shoeing.

However I can't feel too guilty, as later that year, George tried to kill me. In December, we were playing away on another Wednesday evening after work. Slip out early, meet at Euston for an evening match against Coventry, 7.30 kick-off at Coundon Road. We get there, it's freezing and the ground is rock hard. We play a truncated, tentative game, which we lose, catch the 9.30 train home with a few crates and do some rubbish singing.

For some reason, to the tune of 'Onward Christian Soldiers' (today, of course, sung in the bowdlerised twenty-first-century version 'Onward Christian Pilgrims' so as not to cause offence, other than to those who are spinning in their graves), I start singing, 'Lloyd-Roberts knew Prince Charles, Prince Charles knew Lloyd-Roberts, Lloyd-Roberts knew Prince Charles, Prince Charles knew Lloyd-Roberts,' etc. Not very difficult words, even for A.K. Rodgers.

George, who was sitting next to me, smiled from about

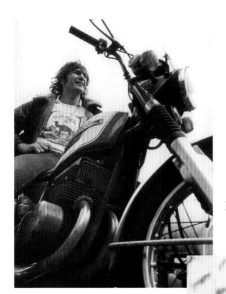

Me aged 25. This is how I still
think of myself – dream on!
(© Don Morley)

England v. Wales, 1974.
Scoring a try under the
posts at Twickenham.
(© E. D. Lacey)

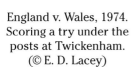

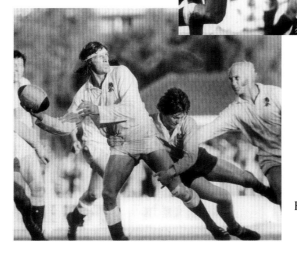

England v. Australia, 1975.
We won that one too.

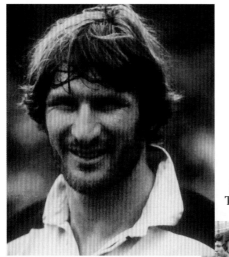

Playing for the Barbarians in 1982.
They loved to run the ball – so did I.

At Paris Université Club.
Gérard Krotoff is in a tie, I'm not.
(© Presse 'E Sports)

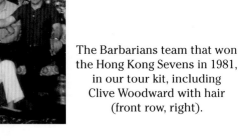

The Barbarians team that won
the Hong Kong Sevens in 1981,
in our tour kit, including
Clive Woodward with hair
(front row, right).

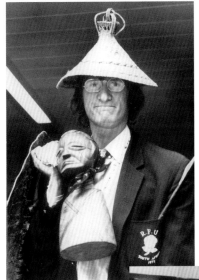

On tour with England in
South Africa, 1972. Every
manager's nightmare.

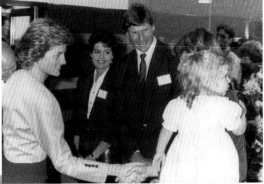

Elisabeth says hello to
Princess Di, late '80s.

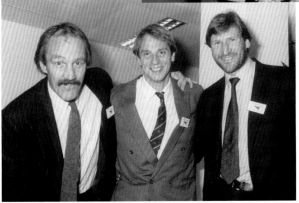

When we were fab.
Big Rog Uttley and
Steve Redgrave and me.

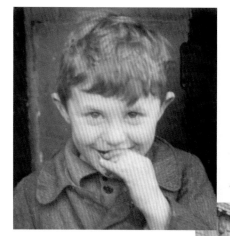

Aged three –
a little Scouser.

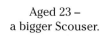

Aged 23 –
a bigger Scouser.

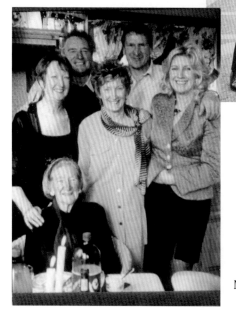

Mum, Jackie, Lois, Eileen,
Mick and myself on
Mum's 90th birthday, 2000.

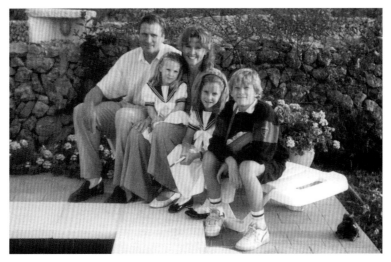

Family man. The way we were in 1989.

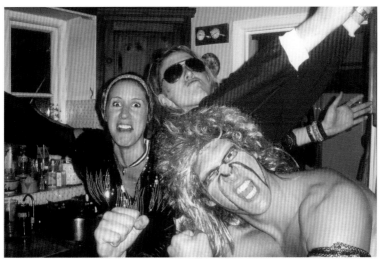

Kids! The way they are – dressing up for dinner in 2007.

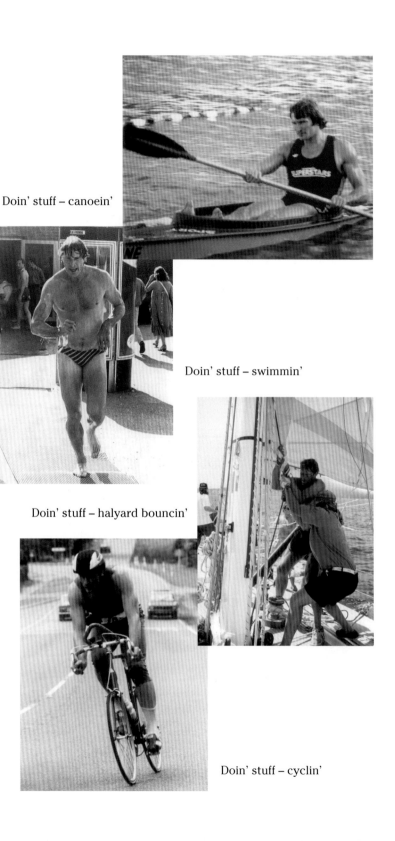

Doin' stuff – canoein'

Doin' stuff – swimmin'

Doin' stuff – halyard bouncin'

Doin' stuff – cyclin'

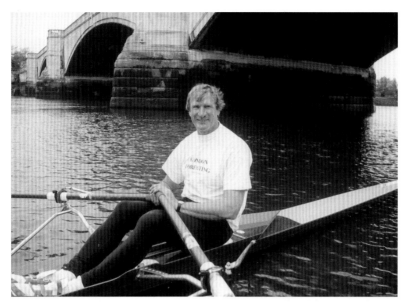

Sculling on the Thames at Chiswick in 2005.

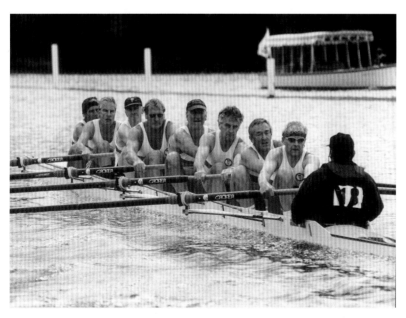

Tideway Scullers School Veteran Eight winning at Henley, 2005.
Three of us had prostate problems. None of us knew.

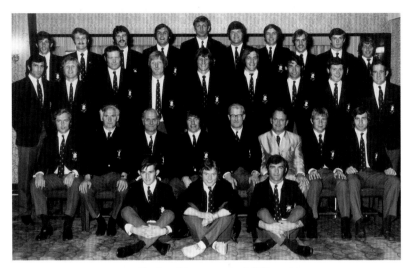

England tour party, 1972.

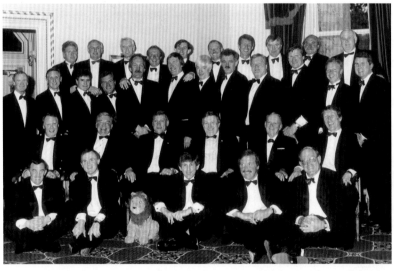

British Lions 1974 reunion, 20 years later. (© Pat McGuigan Photography)

Coventry to about Rugby. By about St Albans we were all really getting into the song: it might have been repetitive, but it was strangely compulsive, in part because George had indeed gone to school with Prince Charles and because, apparently, George's dad had been gynaecologist to the Queen Mother.

Out of the corner of my eye, I just saw a fist. I moved my head, and George hit the glass panel behind my head with such force that the noise was louder than the singing. The singing stopped, nobody said anything, my nose was still where it should be, George would later get medical attention for his hand. Then the small, musically challenged voice of A.K. Rodgers gave us a solo of 'Lloyd-Roberts knew Prince Charles', and by Watford we were all back in full voice again.

I'd come across George again in a quite different field a few years later. In 1986, when I was in my banking pomp, the house I had bought on a mortgage a few years earlier had inexplicably and with absolutely no effort on my part risen in value. Banks would offer me letters of credit based on the fortuitous rise in my property value and I had somehow confused a bull market with brains. I decided to become a name at Lloyd's of London. (A 'name' at Lloyd's is an individual who underwrites insurance, providing the financial backing that acts as security for the policies.) My eyes were wide open, but the decision was driven by the thought of endless cheques gushing through my door for no work. The fruits of capitalism. I had risen from Greenway Comprehensive School, with a rugby ball tucked under my arm, to vertically integrate myself into a place my hard-working mother and father had never been. At Lloyd's, the very nice group of men in the large room with the enormous chandelier and massive boardroom table had told me that if this went wrong,

I could lose everything. They actually said 'down to your last cufflink'. This was unlimited liability.

Did they think I was stupid? I had sat professional exams, served my articles with Price Waterhouse in the City, had postgraduate degrees in finance from the academically prestigious London School of Economics. How could I not know what unlimited liability was? Pride, fall.

George was an underwriter, so I went to him to get some guidance. He went through the detail and process with me. As I was at the door, he said, in a throwaway manner and with great perception, the smartest thing he's ever said to me: 'Andrew, remember you came to me.'

This post-war baby-boom generation has lived through a period of unbelievable privilege, wealth through technological innovation, a sort of freedom and democracy, a sustained period of peace, health, education and choice. Only now, at the beginning of the twenty-first century, are we seeing the cirrus clouds of change high in the sky, if we care to look for them. But right now, Peter Townshend's generation have a degree of choice that was never available to any other generation. Now, in our mid- to late fifties, we have options that were denied to our parents.

George and Lizzie had been married (two children – I'm one of Henry's godfathers) since I had known them. Lizzie wanted to be happy (personally, I blame HRT), and she wasn't with George. She left him to find happiness. George did two things.

First, having scissored half his assets to Lizzie and fearful of an impoverished old age, he worked harder at his trade than at any time in his life.

The second I still find most bizarre. We were, for some reason, sitting having a coffee in one of those restaurants by the lake in St James's Park. George, who had been bashed by the turn of events and had moved out of the family home, was saying that it was the fact that their history had been lost forever that was one of the most difficult things to bear. The other was living alone. He couldn't do it, so he had a plan.

This was George's plan: having, albeit belatedly, taken to computers and spreadsheets, he was going to construct a spreadsheet to find a new woman in his life. I told him this was not the strategy employed, as far as I knew, by Romeo or Eros, with his random arrows of fate. George said that, quite frankly, he had had enough of the random arrows of fate. We had another coffee.

His strategy was to put along the Y-axis a carefully weighted series of factors as to what he wanted from his new precious. Things like she had to be over 50; she had to be either divorced or a widow; she had to be, however remotely, already known to him. Children were a positive. It was quite a long list, and it seemed he had, for whatever reasons, given a lot of thought to it. Along the X-axis he would put in the names of all the women he knew.

He told me he had come up with two names. He had already contacted Jane and told her about the spreadsheet and that she'd sort of won and asked whether he could, having done the spreadsheet and all the hard work, now come and live with her. Jane ventured the opinion that while this approach had something to commend it, it was a bit lacking in romance. She suggested lunch instead.

I don't think he ever contacted the other potential winner, and he and Jane have been together now for three years. She lives in Islington and he lives in the New Forest, but they spend most of the time together, somewhere. When we arrive to visit him, he is alone.

Elisabeth and I get there late, and we all go out for lunch in the village pub. George is a bit like me, wants the world to love him, and the pub does. We have a nice afternoon.

What do I learn about myself? Nothing, but I'm having a nice day.

We drive on to Winchester to meet Chris Keen for dinner. Chris lives in the north part of the New Forest but has rented a house in Winchester during term time so he can travel to London and his children (eight, eleven and thirteen) can walk to school.

We get to Winchester and find a hotel – it's a nice hotel in the centre of the town – park the car and go to reception. We are, apparently, what are called walk-ins. Without prompting, they offer us a deal: double bed for the night and full English breakfast for the same price as the fine for parking in a no-parking area. Yes, please. They also ask us to pay upfront; walk-ins can apparently be walk-outs. The centre of Winchester is worth looking round, as is the abbey. It is sunny. I am in love with Elisabeth.

What did we all do before mobile phones? We arrange to meet Chris off the train from London. Chris is an only child. His father died when he was nine, and Chris was sent away to school. We met in the summer of 1981, when I took a job in the United Bank of Kuwait, a Kuwaiti consortium bank based in Lombard Street in the City. I was appointed with Ralph Halbert (Eton, Oxford and the Guards), both of us as assistant general managers, to diversify the bank's interests. Chris was the deputy general manager, about 30, a natural dealer, sharp, detached, unmarried, known as 'the Ice Man'.

Before I took that job, I had worked in the head offices of Midland Bank, Citibank and the Hungarian International Bank. A hired gun. For the last two years, I'd been at the Hungarian International Bank, working for the general manager, Jack Wilson. My job had been to assess the sovereign risk and bank guarantees on trade finance paper bought by the bank. This meant travelling to South-east Asia, Eastern Europe, the USSR, North Africa and anywhere else they cared to send me and then checking out private and state banks and perceived country risks – potential problems specific to a given nation. It was fun. I also liked sport. In November 1981, although I'd used up all my holiday leave, I was due to go to Hong Kong to compete in the final of *World Superstars*, so I applied for a week's unpaid leave.

Jack called me into his office: 'No problem, and I appreciate what you've done for us, but, Andrew, you've got to decide: do you want to commit yourself to the bank and make some money or be a sportsman?' It was all very amicable, and I would work for Jack again about ten years later, but I decided that I'd spend the next two months swimming, cycling, paddling about on a hired rowing boat on Battersea Lake, running and pistol shooting. Strange, really, as Elisabeth was about to have our first child, the Mouse.

Actually, he is called Marcus. I wanted to call him one of those cowboy names like Joe or Chip, but being present at the birth and seeing the pain involved in it, I thought, Elisabeth, you can call him whatever you like. So Marcus it was, because it also works in German, as do Claudia and Stefanie.

As I said, seeing Marcus's birth and witnessing what Elisabeth went through put all my travails on *Superstars* into perspective; but, hey, don't get me wrong – *Superstars* is the second most painful thing after childbirth.

Superstars was really just garbage TV, perhaps even the trailblazer for all these reality TV shows that pollute our screens today. My God, perhaps I'm in some way responsible for *Celebrity Big Brother*! But back in the early 1970s, when it began, there wasn't much in the way of choice in entertainment for kids. No games consoles, no

Internet and only three television channels. So TV was a huge medium, and families sat round in the evening watching the same programme – which, for about ten years, seemed usually to be *Superstars*.

I'd never been recognised on the street for my rugby exploits, but the moment I appeared on *Superstars*, I couldn't even pop down my local Marks & Spencer's without being mobbed. OK, so that's a slight exaggeration, but you know what I mean. 'Here, aren't you that bloke off *Superstars* what does the rowing and the running?' Being a natural-born attention seeker, I loved it and milked it for all it was worth. The strangest spin-off, however, from my *Superstars* fame was the number of journalists who arrived on my front doorstep wanting my opinion on a wide range of subjects that really I knew nothing about. Still, who was I to complain? I got a free lunch out of it, and they filled their copy for the next day's paper with my thoughts on the cost of a pint of milk.

I'd been as glued to *Superstars* as the rest of the country when it first appeared on the BBC in 1973. I suppose if you were to ask the '*Superstars* generation' now what most sticks out in their minds from its heyday, they would mention Kevin Keegan falling off his bike in 1976 and getting back on, bloodied but unbowed, or perhaps the orange-chomping Brian Jacks on the dips bar. What's been forgotten is the number of world-class athletes who competed at the peak of their powers. As well as people like Keegan (and don't forget, when he fell off his bike he was rated the best footballer in England; I mean, can you imagine the number of puppies Alex Ferguson would have if Wayne Rooney took a tumble appearing on *Superstars* 2007!) and Jacks, who'd won a medal for Britain in judo at the 1972 Olympics, there were guys like Alan Minter, the undisputed middleweight boxing champion of the world, Daley Thompson, Olympic gold medallist in the decathlon, Andy Irvine, Scotland and Lions full-back, and James Hunt, Formula One champion.

When I got a phone call asking me to appear in the 1981 series, I was delighted. I reckoned me and *Superstars* were made for each other. I loved all sports, and as a kid I'd tried my hand at most things – canoeing, athletics, basketball, football. I just loved to run around anyway! And as I soon found out, if you've been coached in a sport as a child, even for a short amount of time, it's amazing how quickly it comes back to you and how just a basic bit of instruction can help.

I was invited to a heat in Peterborough, and from the moment I arrived, I loved it. It was a bit like a glorified school sports day in a way, and my approach was similar to the one I'd used in school exams: I'd give off an air of nonchalance and indifference, but in fact I'd be busting every gut in my body to succeed! I think that was the attitude of all the competitors, because it was all very jokey and laid back . . . until the starter's gun went, and then the competitive animal roared from deep within us all.

One of the great things about *Superstars* was the commentary provided by Ron Pickering and David Vine. Their professionalism dressed it up and lent it a touch of gravitas otherwise absent from ten blokes wearing very tight shorts and sporting very bad haircuts.

There were eight events in each heat, and you had to compete in six of the eight. From the start, I knew I had an advantage over some of my rivals, because the rules stated that you weren't allowed to compete in your own sport. So, for instance, a sprinter wasn't allowed to race the 100 m, and a cyclist had to sit out the bike ride. As a rugby player, I didn't have a 'specialised subject'. (In fact, thinking about it, some of my old teammates and coaches might be shaking their heads at this moment and thinking, 'Andy, rugby wasn't even your specialised subject.')

If you came first in an event you were awarded ten points, second would receive seven, third would get four, fourth two and fifth one point. Got that? Good. Let me tell you, some of the more intellectually challenged superstars never quite understood the scoring system.

I'll be honest and say I can't now recall who was in that first heat in Peterborough, but I do remember powering to victory in the canoeing on the Rive Nene and not doing too badly in the 100 m and the 800 m. The event I always sat out was the gym test, because a 6 ft 6 in. man who weighs 250 lbs is never going to rock the world when it comes to dips and squat thrusts. They're best left to the likes of Brian Jacks.

I won my heat and so made it into the British final, where I lined up against seven other sportsmen, most of whom were infinitely better known than me. Among them were Mick Channon, the former England striker, who was then playing for Southampton; Peter Bonetti, who a year or two before had retired as Chelsea goalkeeper, after making more than 700 appearances; Jim Fox, who'd won a pentathlon gold at the 1976 Olympics; Lynn 'The Leap' Davies, long jump gold medallist at the 1964 Olympics; and David Jenkins, a gold medallist in the 400 m in the European Championships and an Olympic finalist in 1980.

Just about the only bloke who was as unknown as me was Keith Fielding, a rugby-union winger who had switched to rugby league with Salford and represented England at both codes. In fact, when I made my England debut against Wales in 1972, Keith had been on the left wing. He played a couple more times that season and then turned professional. He was a nervous, edgy character and took *Superstars* as seriously as I did, only, unlike me, he was honest enough to show it.

As it turned out, Keith and I finished first and second. I would like to say I was robbed, but I wasn't. Keith was lightning quick and he edged me out in the 100 m to become *Superstars* champion 1981.

Keith and I were subsequently invited to compete in the 1981 *World Superstars*, held, as they always were, in the States. The world version had been held since 1977, and I think the intention had been to invite a few sacrificial non-Americans to be slaughtered on the altar of US dominance. Unfortunately, the organisers' plan backfired. Assuming that the rest of the sporting world was inferior to American athletes, the organisers insisted that the winners of British, Irish, Dutch, etc. *Superstars* had not only to win their own country's competition but also to win a *European Superstars* event to qualify for the world contest. Of course, what this meant was that we few, we happy few, who made it through the qualification process were the very best, because we had come through such a tough and gruelling filtering process. (Brian Budd, a Canadian soccer player, had won *World Superstars* in 1980, and our own Brian Hooper triumphed in 1982.)

The thought of competing against Americans made me even more demented than normal, and I took to splashing about on Battersea Lake in a pathetic attempt to improve my rowing. What had started as a bit of fun had now become some sort of athletics Holy Grail to me. At the age of 33, I really should have known better. Perhaps most damning of all, I even did a bit of homework on my American rivals to find out their strengths and weaknesses. Thinking about it, however, perhaps it wasn't just my competitive streak that made me rise at 6 a.m. to row across Battersea Lake;

the thought of the $35,000 for the winner made the alarm clock easier to obey.

There were eleven superstars in the world final, including Keith Fielding and me from Britain; Declan Burns, an Irish kayaker; Jody Scheckter, the South African racing driver who had won the Formula One world championship in 1979; and Gaétan Boucher, a Canadian speedskater whom I'd never heard of. (But come on, how many North Americans in 1981 knew (a) who Andy Ripley was; (b) what rugby was; and (c) where England was?) The other six competitors were American, including Ann Meyers, a female basketball player, who that year had won the first ever American *Women Superstars*. I've no doubt Ann was a great athlete, but it was an odd decision to include her against ten of the best male sports stars in the world. To her credit, she came fifth in the swimming and third in the football test, but she still finished last by some distance in the overall standings.

Of the Americans, about the only one we Brits had heard of was Edwin Moses, the superb 400-m hurdler, without doubt the greatest exponent of that particular distance in the history of athletics. He'd won gold at the 1976 Olympics in a world-record time of 47.63 sec. and would have retained his title had the USA not boycotted the 1980 games. As it was, he won gold in the 1984 Olympics, and between 1977 and 1987, he won 122 consecutive races in the 400-m hurdles, a phenomenal achievement that makes my personal best of 53.69 sec. look positively snail-like. He was also a very nice bloke.

The other Americans came from American football, basketball, speedskating and track and field. I'd identified the greatest threat as being Russ Francis, a big strong footballer with the New England Patriots. Russ had also been a handy junior athlete and was on a year's sabbatical from the Patriots, a sign of how seriously he was taking *World Superstars*. He reminded me a bit of the Incredible Hulk – just not quite as green.

Peter Mueller, the speedskater who had won gold in the 1976 Winter Olympics, was likely to be my biggest threat in my strongest event, the rowing, but, then again, I kept telling myself, it was unlikely that Mueller had spent weeks training on Battersea Lake. He'd probably had better things to do.

The event was held in Key Biscayne, Florida, and it soon became clear that the organisers were desperate for Russ Francis to win because he was the most marketable. A handsome hunk in a sexy and macho sport, Russ was a marketing man's dream, and *Superstars* wanted a piece of the pie.

Unlike British *Superstars*, in which there were eight events, the world competition had ten disciplines: tennis, the gym test, a 50-m swim, weightlifting, a 100-m row, a 100-m sprint, football shooting, an 800-m run, an obstacle course and a mile cycle. I gave tennis a miss (too uncoordinated) and the dreaded gym test a wide berth.

Surprisingly, Jody Scheckter shot into an early lead, winning the tennis and coming second in the gym test behind Declan Burns. Jody, like the crafty, cunning driver he was, had decided to play the Americans at their own game as far as gamesmanship was concerned, and before the gym test he coated the soles of his trainers with oil. Lo and behold, he whistled off 88 squat thrusts in a minute as his feet slid effortlessly up and down. The nearest Jody ever came to admitting he might have, ahem, used an illegal substance in the gym test was when, after the competition, he plaintively said to me, in such a way that for the first and only time I felt what it must be like to be a

Catholic priest at confession, 'Andrew, let me tell you: I'm short, I'm South African and I'm Jewish – I've got to bend the rules!' I haven't seen Jody since, but he was a top man with whom I got on very well.

So after the first four events, Jody was leading with 24 points, then came Russ Francis with 21, and Declan Burns was third with 14 points. I was joint last with 2 points, which I'd squeezed out of the swim. Faced with the prospect of total and utter humiliation, and the possibility of spending the rest of my days hiding out in shame in the Florida Everglades as a result, I gave the rowing everything I had and a little bit more.

I came first over the 100-m course in a time of 34.97 sec., smashing the existing *Superstars* record by nearly 2 sec. Phew! At least I had made double figures on the scoreboard. In the 100-m sprint, I came third and Keith Fielding came second. Both of us finished about 50 m behind Ed Moses, who'd been allowed to compete even though one might have argued that, as a 400-m hurdler, sprinting came under his 'specialised sport'. But I don't wish to appear a sore loser, bitter and twisted more than a quarter of a century later . . . can you hear that? It's the sound of my teeth being gnashed!

I did better in the other track event, the 800 m, the penultimate event, coming first in a time of 1 min 56.9 sec. and collecting 10 more points. As I failed to trouble the scorers in the obstacle course, I finished *World Superstars* on 27 points, 8 behind Jody Scheckter, the champion, and 4 short of Declan Burns in second spot. But I was the best of the Brits, edging out Keith by 2 points. In fact, I had tied for third with Russ Francis, so we shared $15,600 for our efforts, although I think it's probably fair to say that I was happier with my lot than Russ, who had to return to the NFL saddled with the ignominy of having been beaten in

World Superstars by a short South African and a Paddy paddler!

I have to confess that at the time I was mortified that I hadn't won, despite the insouciant exterior. I like winning! In hindsight, however, I'm glad I didn't, because if I had, I would have kept the $35,000. Under the rules at the time, that would have meant I'd turned professional, and I would no longer have been allowed to play rugby union. As it was, it wasn't long before I received a friendly call from the RFU secretary, Robin Prescott, who, for some odd reason, was a keen follower of mine when it came to *Superstars*. I thanked Robin for his support and asked him whether the RFU would care for a donation of $15,600 for the players' benevolent fund. 'Oh, Andy, how generous.' Still, I'm sure they put the money to better use than I would have, and everyone in the RFU thought I was a brilliant bloke. Which, of course, I am.

My last foray into the increasingly surreal world of *Superstars* was in 1983 for a 'past masters' competition. A case of flogging a dead horse? If only we had shown as much energy as a dead horse during that weekend. It was held at High Wycombe Sports Centre (proof that by now my burgeoning television career knew no bounds) and involved, among others: Lynn Davies (41), Ron Clarke (47), Emlyn Hughes (35), David Hemery (39), Ken Buchanan (38), David Duckham (37), Alan Ball (37) and me, a mere stripling at 35.

I couldn't remember much about the weekend even shortly afterwards, and I can remember even less now. One thing does stick in my mind, though, and it still breaks my heart when I think of it. It was a very social occasion, and all of us got on really well together, even little Kenny Buchanan, who was a fiery Scottish pugilist with an accent so strong and so incomprehensible to a Sassenach that I often found myself just nodding in agreement with whatever he said. We all knew of Ken's reputation as one of the greatest of all British boxers and one of the world's best lightweight fighters, and we also knew that in recent times life had been tough. Not long after his retirement from the ring in the late 1970s, his wife had left him and his hotel business had collapsed, forcing him to return to carpentry, a trade he'd learned before he became a professional boxer.

But Ken took part with his head held high, and he was just a lovely, lovely man. Everywhere he went during the filming of *Superstars: The Past Masters* he carried under his arm something wrapped in a brown paper bag. Eventually, one of us plucked up the courage to ask what it was. 'It's a typewriter,' Ken told us proudly. The full story was that since his divorce, he hadn't seen much of his daughter, but it was her birthday soon; he'd asked her what she'd like and she'd said a typewriter. She and her mum lived quite close to High Wycombe, so she'd promised to visit her dad during the weekend, which is why Ken was carrying the present about under his arm.

But she never showed. At the end of the weekend, I gave Ken a lift to Heathrow for his flight to Scotland. At the airport, he handed me the typewriter and said, 'Here, Andy, you might as well keep this.' A while later, I read that Ken was boxing in unlicensed fights just to earn a couple of hundred quid. Fortunately, he's subsequently got his life back on course. Sadly, though, two of those competitors from *Past Masters* in 1983 are no longer with us. Rest in peace, Emlyn and Alan.

In between rowing on Battersea Lake and practising my television pout in front of the mirror, I was seeking gainful employment. One Thursday, I spotted an advert in the *Financial Times*: 'Banking in East Croydon and California.

Stanford Research Institute have an office in East Croydon and are looking to recruit staff to help with a project for the Midland Bank, who plan to reconfigure the branch network organisation for the next 20 years.'

So in 1981, I found myself in an office at Stanford Research Institute, Menlo Park, Silicon Valley, California. Not that I knew it then, but the whole computer-technology revolution was happening around me. I'm sitting in this room in my suit, 'cause that's what you wear if someone is buying your time, when three Californians in Hawaiian shirts drift in eating stuff. Then the door opens and in comes Ty Auer, Mr California. 'Look, our clients have gotta problem, we don't know much about the problem, it could be a purple cloud. We don't know how big it is or how dense but we've gotta catch that problem, anyone got any ideas?' Assuming this is some sort of joke or a test, before anyone else can speak, I say, 'Ty, have you thought about a brown paper bag?' Ty leaps up and says, 'Andy I just love the way you think!'

Maybe I should have been more adventurous, but a month or two later, I'd said goodbye to California and was saying hello to Chris Keen at the United Bank of Kuwait (UBK), Lombard Street, London. I was nearly ten years working in Lombard Street. At some stage, Chris got made general manager and I got bumped up the hierarchical ladder as well.

The 1980s was a great time to be working in a consortium bank in London. UBK was owned by a number of Kuwaiti banks which were each owned by a family, and they just let the British management get on with running the bank. They assumed we wouldn't steal from them, and we assumed they trusted us; the four or so board meetings a year in London or Kuwait were very gentlemanly affairs. The Bank of England kept an eye on everyone in the background.

Corporate governance and regulation with teeth were still ten years away. This was before the development of Canary Wharf, and the City was the hub of the financial world, with everything concentrated in the area around the Bank of England. The Stock Exchange and the Baltic shipping exchange were still thriving markets in which deals were done face to face (today, most of their business is done online), there was the emerging futures market and Lloyd's new building, and all these were surrounded and enhanced by a proliferation of foreign banks, clearing banks, merchant banks and the associated legal and accounting services, gyms and restaurants. The world was awash with Eurodollars and the new technology and opportunity. 'My word is my bond' was a principle that still operated to some extent in the City, and it was not so far from the Kuwaiti view: 'It is in the heart and eyes that deals are made.' This comfortable world was to be rocked by a number of scandals, but in the early '80s, this was Fun Street.

I can remember on one occasion in Kuwait standing outside the Public Institute Social Security (I kid you not, although someone did eventually put in an 'of') and asking the official if we could increase the bank's equity from £30 million to £60 million, which would allow us to borrow £600 million to grow the bank. It seemed like asking for a resident's parking permit in Fulham – it was simply no big deal.

Kuwait was awash with oil revenue and wanted to become the Switzerland of the Gulf. With an indigenous population of about half a million and twice as many foreign workers – Lebanese, Iraqi, Palestinian, Indian, British, etc. – there was a degree of xenophobia, but this was directed largely against other Arabs, who tended to see the Kuwaitis as the pools winners of the region. The real heart of Arab culture was in Cairo, Damascus, Amman or Baghdad, not in Kuwait City. In fact, the idea of an Arab nation seemed ludicrous – they all disagreed on almost everything, except for their dislike of Israel.

With Chris, I also witnessed, at first hand and in the raw, how an unregulated kerbside market works. The Kuwait government, with the best of intentions (that of recirculating the excess oil cash to stimulate the economy), gave land to each of its indigenous citizens and then bought the land back. It was hoped that this cash windfall would fund the entrepreneurial zeal of those citizens. It didn't; it gave the players the stake money for the Soukh al Manack.

The Soukh al Manack was a shopping mall with lots of boutiques selling gold, or at least that's what it started out as. It became, instead, a shopping mall of financial dreams and aspirations. Kuwait consists of a number of tribes and, within those tribes, families. Traditionally, the menfolk would meet in the evening after the sun had gone down and sit, drink tea and talk over issues or plans in the *diwaniyah*, the male social hub of the family.

So, in 1981, this is how it happened in the diwaniyah: Anwar might say he intends to set up a company with, for example, the exclusive Mercedes truck sales franchises in Kuwait and Basra. He is going to raise equity capital by issuing 100,000 ordinary shares at 2 dinars per share. Bashir says he would like to buy for 20,000 dinars 10,000 ordinary shares, and he writes a six-month post-dated cheque payable to the company for 20,000 dinars. The only rule of this market is that foreigners should not be allowed in to rip the Kuwaitis off.

At this point, Hamed might go to Anwar and ask if he can buy some shares. Anwar says, look, the company hasn't been set up yet, we aren't trading, and I don't want to sell shares in something that doesn't exist, but ask Bashir.

Bashir agrees to sell 5,000 ordinary shares to Hamed but at 4 dinars per share on a six-month post-dated cheque.

Bashir now has a future obligation of 20,000 dinars and a future revenue of 20,000 dinars and 5,000 ordinary shares in this company for which he is now being offered 10 dinars per share. Get the idea? It was financial mayhem.

The diwaniyahs moved into the shopping boutiques of the Soukh al Manack; the gold traders moved out: they couldn't compete. The speed with which this market picked up was massive, limited only by the ability of an individual to write a cheque. There was free entry and exit to the Soukh, even to foreigners. Chris and I went in and were swept away by the pace, the energy. It was rumoured that the urinals in the Soukh had been sold for 5 million US dollars. You could not help but be swept up in the tidal wave of not greed exactly but excitement, fever, even if you weren't in any way involved. Paper wealth was being created at such a rate that when eventually the house of cards did fall, post-dated cheques had to be met even prior to due date if presented in Kuwait. One Kuwaiti customs official had obligations in excess of 16 billion dollars, more than the entire Polish national debt at that time.

The reverberations were to be felt throughout the Gulf for many years and what was in a man's heart and eyes was replaced, sadly, by teams of lawyers getting everything signed in triplicate.

UBK allowed me to earn a livelihood and play sport and make friends. I think all of us who worked in that place look back on it with great fondness. It couldn't last. The Kuwaitis wanted to run what was theirs, the stock market crash of 1987 left the British management vulnerable and rugby had given me up, so I decided to set myself up in a few ventures, some of which Chris got involved in, if only for old times' sake. He then, at the age of 50, retired from UBK and carried on trading. He had got married at the age of about 40 (which was great – otherwise he would have become a crusty old grump) to Tamsyn, who is 12 years younger.

Chris came to visit me in East Surrey Hospital with his three young children. He knows how it is; he had a triple heart bypass nine years ago.

We meet and eat. We have a nice evening. What do I learn about myself? Nothing, but I'm still having a nice day.

Tuesday, 18 October 2005

(but written on 7 November 2005)

We drive up the A34 to Oxford, pick up some sailing stuff before heading back down via East Ilsey towards Cornwall and dropping in on Nick Watkins, who is married to Gillie and, like Chris, has three young children. I'd forgotten that people still have to work, like every day. Gillie gives me a plate of mulligatawny soup. Her lovely mum died suddenly of pancreatic cancer; blink and she was gone, just six weeks from diagnosis to death. Her dad, Stormin' Norman, is a walking miracle. He should have turned up his toes long ago but is still in there. There is such an unfair randomness about cancer: Darwin's merciless world of random cruelty.

Along the M4 down the M5. Maybe it was the late night the night before or the travel or dehydration, but whatever the reason, Elisabeth and I have a row. Sometimes you have a row, it just comes out of nowhere for no reason and it passes. However, here, there was a reason.

I – don't ask me why, maybe it's insecurity – want to be friends with the world. I want to be friends with people even when I know I'll never see them again. I think this is actually quite a nice characteristic, but for the person you're with, it means you are paying them less attention. In fact, you make more of an effort with the guy at the petrol station than you do with the person who has given you their life.

For four months now, Elisabeth has been like a rock: she has just got on with it, she has been there for me and not made a big deal of anything. One of the great benefits of this cancer stuff is the wonderful kindness I have experienced and been shown. For me, this has been the best and most wonderful side effect of this disease. I am an attention seeker, I do love the spotlight – again, don't ask me why, maybe it's still insecurity. I have become wrapped up in myself; I am having an affair with cancer. Elisabeth has been locked out.

Added to which, we are on the way to meet up with my brother and three sisters. We are close as siblings, always have been. It is difficult, always has been, for our partners, who, I imagine, even if not directly, ask the question, 'Are you with me or are you with them?' Two years ago, at one of these family get-togethers without children and grandchildren that we have every year around the first week of December, Brian, my sister Eileen's husband, asked the seemingly innocuous question, 'Is there a later train?' World War Three broke out. What was it about? Goodness knows, but underlying it was this question, 'Where does your loyalty lie?'

During the car journey, I was angry. About what, I was not too sure. Elisabeth was angry, with reason. We drove to Fowey, a beautiful little port. We left the car in the only car park, out of town, high on the hill. Despite the fact that it was eight o'clock in October and the car park was empty, we still had to pay. We walked down the steep passage. It was quiet and narrow, and I could see then why cars should be dumped outside of town. It was dark on the quayside with, strangely, little moonlight, although there was a spring high tide with all those accompanying noises you get when the water gently laps up to and just over the harbour wall. The magic wasn't working. Neither of us was speaking. We had a wonderful meal, bouillabaisse for two at Sam's. We still weren't speaking.

Why was I so angry? Was it because Elisabeth wouldn't play the game, wouldn't take part in the imaginary popularity contest in which I was involved, because that is not her game, and somehow I felt she should because of my condition? Was I using cancer to guilt-trip her to do what I wanted to do and be what I wanted to be, even though she wanted none of these things? Was I at the moment a completely selfish, self-obsessed, self-interested tosser?

I'd come to find out about myself through friends and family and strangers, and I realised that to achieve that objective, actually I needn't even have left home.

My friends were as they always were and as I know they always will be, and I found that when it came to dealing with my illness, they would take their lead from me. The lady who had said to me in jest, 'Oh no, not another old man droning on about his illnesses,' well, she was right. Better for all concerned to do 'brave and bold'. And yet I can't help but think: even better, how about, Andrew, just be yourself. Whatever that is. As Clouds had shown me on the beach in Kalamata, if you want to do a bit of wallowing in self-pity, well just do it. Family and good friends will cope. If you wanna be the brave little soldier, that's also OK, and if you can't be yourself, brave little soldier is probably the best option.

But there is one caveat to the notion that simply being yourself might be the best way to deal with the situation. Maybe I should be more considerate of the one person who would happily carry me for a while if 133 turned out not to be a mistake and events did follow the course that Mike Swinn had anticipated on 24 June. Maybe I should try to stop being so self-obsessed. Actually, at the moment, this prostate cancer isn't so hard for me: no symptoms, no real side effects – yet. But it is hard on those around me. Maybe I should be a little more sensitive not to the guy in the petrol station, to whom I can still be friendly, but to those who care for me and care about me. We wandered back up the hill.

Perhaps we had been hungry or perhaps the warm October magic of Fowey was now working for us as it has worked for others or perhaps at the age of 57 I was growing up. Often the best part of making up is being close to someone and making love.

A side effect of the Zoladex hormone treatment is a huge reduction in your libido. The pituitary gland, which lies at the base of the brain, controls the production of the male sexual hormone and other hormones. It does this by releasing messenger hormones called follicle-stimulating hormone (FSH) and luteinising hormone (LH). Gonadorelin (gonadotrophin or LHRH) analogues interfere with the production of these hormones. I am still physically able to have erections, and because I still have a functioning prostate, I am still able to produce ejaculate, but I have little interest in sex. I had mentioned this to Brian Sweeney, fellow member of both clubs (Tideway Scullers School and the Prostate Cancer Club), who, at the same time, 24 June, as I was being diagnosed, was being given a radical prostatectomy. His response was, 'Well, I've got the opposite problem at the moment, Andy, lots of libido and not much function.'

I don't know much about love, other than that to love and be loved is just the best thing. I know that, tumbling down the ages, in many languages, and many literatures this same sentiment has been expressed far better by many others, and they are not wrong, but, then again, Billy Boy, neither am I. To love and be loved is a part of the multifaceted answer to that Rubik's Cube puzzle of a question, 'Is this it?'

Being impotent, or having a lack of libido, is quite frankly not a situation in which any man would want to be, and there is no way round that simple statement. To be a man and yet not a man, could, if you let it, be the start of a slippery slope to a lack of self-esteem and/or depression. However, it needn't be that way. There are all sorts of aids and medications, which I feel are not appropriate for me at present, but for others they may be the way forward, or at least part of the way forward. Although one thing is for sure, even if you and your doctors opt for the 'watchful waiting' approach to treatment (non-intervention), and that is that prostate cancer in any shape or form and at any stage, whether you have surgery, radiotherapy, hormone treatment or any combination, is unlikely to enhance the actual mechanics of sex. However, love is not just about the mechanics of sex.

Paradoxically, I feel more loving, more caring and more passionate than at any time in my life. When my daughter hugged me and kissed me and said, 'You can tell me, Dad,' was this just not the finest thing a parent can hope for?

Elisabeth is private and I respect that privacy. I cannot imagine what it is like to be without a partner and how difficult it must be to find a partner if you are impotent. I think, perhaps wrongly, that love can be better and sex can still be a large part of your life, if you want it to be. Communication, physical, mental or emotional, is the key.

Elisabeth and I made up, we did not make love, I didn't

want to, but we were in love, and the next few days were easy.

Well you've gotta meet them sometime, so now is as good a time as any. (This part of my story could be a huge incentive to give up, turn to the end and see what happens to me. Does he get away with it? Or does he die? Hey, kiddos, that's my life you're talking about, and I'm glad I don't know the outcome, because it would mean I'd miss today, and today, now, this moment is the most precious time, as the future is guaranteed to no one.) OK, you know those nineteenth-century Russian novels where you are introduced to twenty characters in the first two pages and spend the rest of the book trying to work out who is who? Well, this is a guide to my family.

Andrew George Ripley (me, 58 on 1 December 2005), married to Elisabeth, three children (Marcus, 24, Claudia, 22, and Stef, 19). My father, George (1902–1986), whom I never saw between the ages of 7 and 22, as my parents separated. My mum, Jessie (1908–2000), was a teacher and devoted her life to us children and grandchildren.

My parents were married in 1937. My father worked in the merchant navy; he was torpedoed three times during the Second World War. Every two years, my father would come home on leave, and they obviously didn't believe in contraception, because every two years, my mum got pregnant. In ascending order: me (58); Eileen (60), married firstly to Keith Harper (two children, Katie and Amelia), then to Brian Bennett (two children, Lucy and Bella); Lois (62), married always to Will Crumpton (four children, Emma, Vicki, Joanne and Tom); Jackie (64), married first to Frank Andoh (two children, Adjoa and Yeofi), then to Donald Whittle. Mick (66), married to Angela (two children, Anna and Matthew).

Mum's fifteen grandchildren are now breeding; I am currently great-uncle to ten children, and if they keep up last year's production rate, it'll be about fifty before they're done. Strangely for my brothers and sisters, we only have one cousin, Geoffrey. At the beginning of the twentieth century, when my parents were born, they were English, white, Anglo-Saxon Protestants. My generation of the family, born in the 1940s, were pretty much the same. The next generation, in this period of wealth, communication, travel and expansion, have happily diversified. As have our children's children. We, as an extended family, now cover most religions, most skin colours, a variety of races and nationalities and various positions on the barometer of affluence. In fact, to date, none of my parents' great-grandchildren are English, white, Anglo-Saxon Protestants. It's great. We're a mess, but we're a British mess. It's great being British, which is a massively inclusive term: you can be English British, Black British, Muslim British, Jewish British, lesbian British, Park Lane British . . . the list could go on and on.

We arrive at Mick and Angela's house, although they are not going to be there till late that night. Lois is there, as is Will. Lo cries when we have family arguments, which makes us all feel very small. If previous such get-togethers are anything to go by, Lo is gonna cry sometime in the next couple of days. Will has been Lo's squeeze since we lived in Bristol in the 1960s. I was still at school when he moved into our three-storey house, plus cellars, near Durdham Downs. Mum rented out the top floor to Mrs Monk, who was very old and had a room next to Will's. Mum had bought the house with her sister, Auntie Leah, whose husband had been scrum-half for Bristol Rugby Club. Uncle Tommy died young, following a stroke, and Auntie Leah lived on the second floor. Auntie Leah, also a teacher (as are just about all the women in my family), was pretty racy: she took Continental holidays, said 'bloody' in front of us children and smoked, lots. She died of lung cancer aged 61. Will was red-haired and practical and took me to buy my first motorbike. He also covered Lois's Fox's Glacier Mints, because I kept stealing them from her bag, with stuff that is meant to stop you biting your nails. It was always a major disappointment to Will that not only didn't I complain, but I probably didn't even care. When you're thirteen and know just about everything that is worth knowing, a Fox's Glacier Mint versus a bit of foul-tasting anti-nail-bite gunk is no contest.

There is now a danger for me in that I imagine everyone over 50 has prostate cancer, and I want to help them. Will, now aged 65, had a PSA test last year (5) and is having another next month. Will is brave and private. The following day, all us siblings and wives and husbands take a trip in the October sun on the ferry from Padstow to Rock to have lunch at the St Enodoc Golf Club, but as the tide is so low, we have a long walk across the narrow estuary from far beach to far beach. Will gets a pain in the base of his spine and pelvis if he has to walk a long way. So I imagine that this is a symptom, that Will might have metastatic prostate cancer, which might have gone outside his prostate and into his spine. I say nothing. For some reason, I fear for other people and in particular, at that moment, for Will. Am I just transferring my own hidden anxieties onto other people? Probably. Will wouldn't want me to say anything. I don't.

Lunch is great. Eileen has had a bungalow facing the Camel Estuary for about five years, with Brian, who was born in Cornwall but is, whatever he says, far more Wimbledon than Cornwall. Eileen actually has houses all over the place. Which is remarkable, as she lives on a shoestring. Jackie and Don are staying with her this year.

We repeat the same midday formula the following day, but going to St Mawes on the south coast: a stroll to the castle at the end of the promontory and then lunch in the Rising Sun. Just ten old people out on a spree, not much happens. Except for this. There is a long inviting table in the bay window, in the sunshine; two men even older than us are sitting there finishing their lunch. The publican does a good take on Mr Grumpy. We all sit at the back. It's grim up north and at the back. The two men leave and Brian moves to make a proprietorial claim on Sunshine Corner. Brian is quick but not quick or Cornish enough to cut off a pre-emptive move by Mr and Mrs Really-Impressively-Quick-on-Their-Feet-at-Their-Age. We watch with resignation Brian's game but futile attempt on our behalf.

Then something nice happens that changes our world. Mr and Mrs RIQOTFATA offer to let us sit in Sunshine Corner. Everybody gets happy, Brian buys everyone a drink, including the very good old RIQOTFATAs. Michael asks them if they can guess who the siblings are and who are the partners. They are really, really good at giving up Sunshine Corner but rubbish at this game. The chef comes in, and she is the antidote to Mr Grumpy, who appears to have gone. Was he just a figment of our imaginations? The food is brilliant, the company is better, it's turning out just fine in Sunshine Corner and grim at the back is now but a faded and distant memory.

Later that evening, Elisabeth drives us both home, as tomorrow morning I've an appointment with a big needle and some more Zoladex.

Saturday, 22 October to Sunday, 30 October 2005

(but written on 7 November 2005)

The morning after that I've another appointment, with a big iron bird, the 6.55 Stansted to Jerez. The impact of cheap flights has been huge: budget companies like Ryanair, easyJet, bmi baby, Condor, etc., coupled with Internet booking, have transformed air travel. Huge savings have been passed on to the customer. Interesting pricing policies mean that if you book ahead, it can be cheaper to get to somewhere abroad than it is to get to the departure airport. If, on the other hand, you travel at school half-term, say, and leave it late and have a fixed destination, then get your chequebook out. Charge? In some circumstances, these same airlines' prices do actually compare to the actions of the noble 600 of the Light Brigade. Still they've gotta make a turn, and even then they are still cheaper than the big national flag carriers.

So, slightly financially bruised, after a flight on a full Ryanaircraft, I arrive in Jerez de la Frontera. In a few years, these airlines have done more for European integration than the myriad of bureaucrats in Brussels have done in 40 years. My fellow passengers seem to be taking late holidays, looking at or buying property, just popping over for the weekend or whatever; and it's two way, as there are about as many Spanish as British people travelling.

It's about 50 km to Cadiz; the bus costs about 2 euros, the taxi 50. I realise that at this stage I am coming over as being mean. Well, I'd like to think that I am with myself but not with friends or family. Also, as I am self-employed, keeping costs down gives me more time to do what I want to do rather than having to work. Added to which, I'm both an accountant by training and of the Mr

Micawber school of economics: weekly income nineteen shillings and sixpence, weekly outgoings twenty shillings, misery; weekly income twenty shillings and sixpence, weekly outgoings twenty shillings, unbounded joy. Well, it's something like that. An alternative approach is that of Winston Churchill: he spent what was necessary to give him the lifestyle he wanted and then hassled around for the revenue to fund that lifestyle. A brave and interesting approach and, I imagine, not dissimilar to that of most bank robbers.

The taxi driver drops me off at Pontoon P, Porto Sherry Marina: mid-morning, nobody about and warm Spanish October sun – just great. There is something romantic about going to a port and looking for the boat you are going to join. Although, for the first time, I am suddenly hit by a really urgent need to pee. There is no lavatory and even if there was, I couldn't make it; I find a corner. Hey, I lived in France for six months and played for and toured with Paris Université Club, and I was there, shocked I might add, when in a nightclub in Noumea, New Caledonia, one of the players peed on the singer. There is a huge difference between Latin and Anglo-Saxon culture (although, to be fair, the singer was rubbish). There is also a difference between a young man being fairly crude and rude and an old man with a sense of urinary urgency. I don't know which is the worse. If I get to be incontinent, it looks like I'll need to do some nifty forward planning, although most of the guys I've spoken to say a catheter isn't so bad. It's just the way it is, or the way it maybe will be for me.

I find the Oyster 47 *Kindness*, which, I mentioned before, is named after Jonathan Shingleton's doctor, Hugh Kindness – what a brilliant name for a doctor, or for anyone, really.

I've met Jonathan for 20 minutes. I've never met the other crew member, Nick Booth, before. Nick is fixing the impeller, whatever that is, and he makes me a cup of tea.

It's going to be good. Nick, in his early 40s, is a natural sailor and probably fell in love with the sea at the same time as he was born. Over the next five days, he was to save our lives every minute of every hour of every day. Jonathan and I go to the local supermarket to pick up provisions. If you're ever in Porto Sherry Marina and go to the nearest supermarket and have a huge trolley of stuff, the best thing you can do to get a taxi is to go into the flower shop opposite the supermarket. There you will find a beautiful young Spanish girl with dark brown eyes who will order you a taxi and throw you a smile that will make your heart soar.

Jonathan, diagnosed positive seven years ago with a PSA of 30, had an almost immediate bad reaction to his hormone therapy and chose not to have surgery but to undergo radiotherapy. He is a successful businessman and, following his treatment, decided to do things, one of which was to compete in the Atlantic Rally for Cruisers (ARC) from Las Palmas in Gran Canaria to St Lucia in the Caribbean in his own sailing boat. I suppose we all have challenges and lists of things to do. For Eric, standing up and walking is his challenge.

Jonathan, having learned how to sail, bought this boat three years ago. He had the idea of filling it with guys who had or had had prostate cancer for the ARC in order to raise funds for the Prostate Research Campaign UK. He also wanted to let prostate-cancer sufferers, particularly those who had just been diagnosed, know that there was always not only hope but the opportunity to keep living life to the full.

There is no wind, so we have an early night, diesel up in the morning and motor off with a slight tail wind in the mainsail, out of Cadiz Bay, where we certainly wouldn't have wanted to be 200 years ago almost to the day – it's right off Cape Trafalgar. From Cadiz to Las Palmas is about 800 miles. We will sail at about 7 knots per hour when the wind is above 15 knots (force 3) and if there is little wind, motor at about 6 knots per hour. We have enough diesel for about 500 miles, but all of us want to sail.

Sailing is brilliant, especially on somebody else's boat. After a few days, the boat becomes your entire universe. Nothing is of such consequence as, say, the next sail change, and your days are built around meals and, at night, being on watch. Days merge into each other. The wind never gets up above gusting 6, although even that is uncomfortable enough on a 30-degree tack heading into Atlantic rollers, particularly if you are trying to sleep in the fo'c'sle.

One of the best bits is the robin that appears out of nowhere. Although we are never closer than 80 miles to the North West African coast, it flies round the boat, sits on the rigging as if it were in a tree in Ho Chee's garden and then just flies off. We also see a pod of about 20 dolphins that jump and dive and surf around the yacht and keep us company for an hour or so. A sea turtle that raises its head as we go past or a couple of random porpoises can make our day.

However, the very best bit is the watch from 11 p.m. to 2 a.m. The other guys are sleeping, it's still 20°C, a good warm breeze is filling up the skyscraping sails that stretch all the way to the white navigation light, Africa is way off to the east, there are no ships. The water is flowing around the boat, the autopilot is holding us on a course of 220 degrees. The moon, with its low trajectory at 30 degrees north, will come up later, but for now it is pitch black. You are lying in the cockpit with your head on the cushions looking up at the cloudless sky. Never have I seen so many stars. Starry, starry sky.

Then again, at times I feel like my children in the back of the car about 15 years ago: when are we going to get there, Dad? At 6 knots per hour, quite some time yet, my little darlings. We are taking the boat to Las Palmas so it can compete in the race, which starts on 22 November. This is Jonathan's dream about to be realised, and Nick sails, it defines him, that's what he does. I am pleased for them, but it doesn't define me, and it isn't my dream.

I am also shocked and grateful to Nick and Jonathan. Why? Because I never realised it before, but my knees are shot to bits; on a rolling boat, getting around is difficult. My halyard-bouncing days may well be over. I do my watches, clean the head and make meals when it is my turn, but going forward to fix the navigation lights in rolling breakers is not what I'm good at. Jonathan and Nick sometimes carry me – well, metaphorically.

Five days out of Cadiz, early morning, we've been able to see the lights of Las Palmas for three or four hours; coming into a harbour is great, as is leaving a harbour. It's just the bit in between which can be both brilliant and not brilliant.

We berth, and I take Jonathan and Nick out for a celebratory breakfast. We've got on well but are probably unlikely to see each other again. We will all get on with our separate and different lives. Was prostate cancer a consideration? Not at all. Jonathan and I didn't talk about it much; it was just something he had had, which he had hopefully moved on from and which I was dealing with. Although it was undoubtedly the reason he was realising a dream and also the reason I was there. What did I find out about myself, other than that my knees are worse than I thought? Not so much. What did they think of me? Well, you'd need to ask them.

More pointless advice: don't go to Las Palmas airport looking to pick up a cheap flight to the UK on All Saint's Sunday, 'cause they don't exist. So I took a flight to Stuttgart care of Condor Airways (the alternative was Kiev), got to Stuttgart at just before midnight, slept in the airport (very *Europe on $5 a Day*), caught a train to Mannheim, another one to Paris and a cheapo flight from Charles de Gaulle to Gatwick. Getting home was almost more adventurous than the sailing.

Tuesday, 15 November 2005

So I'm up to date. Did I find out anything new about myself wandering about amongst close friends, family and people who didn't know me from a bar of soap? Not really. Nothing that Elisabeth couldn't already have told me in five minutes over a bowl of cornflakes.

One other thing did happen during the last couple of weeks: I got momentarily famous. Paul had written a kind article about me in the *Sunday Times* on the day I left Cadiz, and on the way, eventually, through Customs at Gatwick, the passport man, without looking at my passport, said, 'Hello, Andy.' I loved it. I am such a tart.

Also, as a result of the same article, I got invited to speak at the Rugby Writers' Dinner on 16 January 2006, which is the sort of unofficial, informal AGM of world rugby union, lots of different agendas, where the after-dinner speaker habitually dies on his feet awash in a sea of heard-it-all-beforeism. Perhaps this year I can die for real.

I went to see my friend Steve today. He's pretty excited about people with MS getting cannabis on the NHS. I am such a fraud. Lynne gave me another shot of Zoladex, and my INR is steady at 2.7.

I go back to the Marsden in about a month's time. I've been reading up about the mechanics of cancer. I don't know much, but I know more than I did almost five months ago, when I was diagnosed. I'll wait till tomorrow to write about what I've found out.

Wednesday, 16 November 2005

Today and today and today. Gosh, Mr Knee, the English master at Greenway Comprehensive School *circa* 1959 to 1966, would have been proud of me. A schoolboy Shakespearean parody and it ain't even eight o'clock in the morning. I sit here tap-tap-tapping away when I should be out on the river. Can I embrace life if all I do is tap-tap-tap away? When the cry in the street is less than the cry in the book are we, am I, missing the point of it all? Is life there to be lived and not tap-tap-tapped away? Maybe not. Maybe not now, maybe there is a time for living and a time for tapping, and today I'm in the tapping time.

To summarise, where has this tapping got me? God, love, myself, cancer and research.

Research, I know about. You absorb all there is to absorb, then add something new, and if you can objectively prove or disprove the something new, you then move on and leave your twig on the bonfire so that when someone else brighter and smarter than you asks the same question they have more twigs than you had.

God. I know I have a poor Christian faith riddled with rational agnosticism. Am I just too weak to admit faith alone is just not good enough? But this can't be all there is, there has to be a point to life, our lives. Neither am I jealous of those who have faith. Those four young men with rucksacks on their backs at King's Cross station on 7 July, standing together with an unquestioning belief that they would meet again in half an hour in paradise, maybe they could have done with a dose of rational agnosticism to prevent them from wrecking and destroying the innocent. Weren't they scared of what God would say to them?

Love is the best. To love and be loved. Thanks to cancer, I know I am loved.

Myself. I know nothing more than I knew already, and friends, family and strangers will take their lead from you. Value yourself, and your life and every life has value. The usual stuff.

Cancer. Well, today, I've just got two things to write about: one is an observation about how we define and categorise cancer, and the other is a passing comment about treatments for prostate cancer and personal medical agendas. 'Spect you're now on the edge of your seat.

Cancers, all cancers, are traditionally defined by where the primary cancer is located. This is sensible and is the bedrock of cancer treatment, study and research. I fully recognise that merely having a cancer, reading a few books and searching the Internet in no way makes me an expert, and I'm bearing in mind that saying about a little knowledge being a dangerous thing. So what I have to suggest is merely a thought to be discarded, but it is a thought, and this is it.

I believe no one has ever died from cancer in the prostate. What 10,000 men in the UK die from every year is the secondary cancers that spread from the prostate and invade the nerve tissues and then the lymph nodes and the bones.

The body is composed of many billions of cells, more cells than I saw stars on that starry, starry night watch, organised into tissues and organs. Cells have the ability to divide and grow, and after a cell has reached its allotted life span or after injury, it can be replaced exactly by another. Most cells live, grow, divide and die according to a particular pattern. Each cell's entire DNA content is replicated when it divides, and today, in your body, millions of such cell divisions are taking place.

Today and every day, mistakes can be made during this process of cell division, and each day these mistakes are detected and rectified by the body. However, occasionally this does not happen, and a cell develops abnormally. This means cells in a particular area grow in a disorganised or uncontrolled manner, such that these cells bypass the normal control mechanisms. These cells will have their own characteristics, which may or may not be similar to their intended function and life span. These cells and similar companion cells may form lumps or tumours.

Oncology is the study of those tumours. If the cells that make up the tumour show no signs of leaving their companion disorganised cells or attempting to invade other parts of the body, the tumour will be referred to as benign. Not all benign tumours arise because of mistakes during cell division; benign enlargement can also be due to an increase or growth in the number of normal cells. In the prostate, this enlargement can be due to a normal growth in the number of cells (BPH). A benign tumour should not be life threatening, although if it is growing in a restricted space, for example in the skull or the prostate, while it will not invade the surrounding tissues, it may physically press against other organs, with consequent side effects. Marcus Rose's brain tumour is an example, as are urinary concerns associated with BPH.

If a cell has certain characteristics such that it will invade areas outside its normal location, this will result in the local advancement of the tumour, and it is said to be malignant. This is cancer, and it will be defined by the initial location of the malignant tumour, not by the characteristics of the invading rogue cell. Why? Because those characteristics are themselves very difficult to define. The pathologist will look at the biopsy sample under a microscope and give an informed view on the aggressiveness of the tumour (which will be reflected in the Gleason score). Even then, though, it is only a view, and it is unlikely that the nature of the rogue cells can really be pinned down. So rogue cells are defined by their location in the body. The character of the rogue cell and its ability to replicate will control the growth of the tumour and its spread. Besides invading, the other characteristic of malignant cells is to set up colonies, or 'seed' themselves, in more remote parts of the body. This metastatic growth results in the formation of secondaries. These colonies will continue to grow in size and number and will damage normal cells in the surrounding areas.

So cancer is rogue cells that have bypassed the normal control mechanisms. These cells will have certain traits or characteristics. They will/may grow by cell division and will/may invade and advance locally and will/may metastasise to distant parts of the body. Why the 'will/may' caveat? Because the nature of the cancer is a function of the characteristics of the rogue cell. One hundred British men will be told today that they have prostate cancer, but that is all they will have in common. Each one of them/us will have their/our own bespoke cancer, which will act according to the characteristics of the rogue cells. For example, it is possible that my tumour has cells which produce large amounts of PSA but are not aggressive or invasive. Dream on, Andrew. It is possible that another man may have cells that produce little PSA but are invasive. We may all have prostate cancer, but each one of us has our very own bespoke variety. Lucky us.

This clearly makes the detection of cancer, definition of the stage it has reached and its treatment difficult. However, even if we have our own bespoke diseases, it is also the case that empirical observation and the associated experience have identified common patterns, and it is around these common patterns that most diagnoses and treatments are hung.

This is just an observation about how we define and categorise cancer. I place my unimpressive twig on the bonfire. The next thing I have to say is a comment about treatments for prostate cancer and personal medical agendas.

So, using my twig, what I've learned so far is that although every cancer is bespoke, each cancer is identified by where it originates in the body. This is a pragmatic approach but it should never be forgotten that your prostate cancer will have the characteristics of the rogue cell that first created the tumour. I might be diagnosed as having prostate cancer, but each prostate cancer will have the characteristics specific to the rogue cell that has created the invasive tumour. Empirical observation has identified a probable basic growth pattern of prostate cancer, which is early cancer (tumour in the prostate) to locally advanced cancer (tumour expanded through the prostate membrane) to metastatic cancer (the rogue cells have seeded themselves in distant sites). There are a series of far more sophisticated and convoluted gradings. However, this is not a priori how your cancer will necessarily progress; that will depend on the rogue cells' characteristics.

There are five methods of treatment – watchful waiting, surgery, radiotherapy, hormone treatment and alternative/

complementary therapies – each with a variety of subsets and each with a range of potential short- and long-term effects. These treatments are not mutually exclusive, indeed they are often more effective when used in some combination.

A potential issue is this: we have a bespoke cancer that is defined pragmatically by its physical location, not by its characteristics, at which we can only make a guess, albeit an informed guess based on observation. Added to which, that cancer may be at any point along a continuum from being contained in the prostate to having spread to distant sites.

There is ample scope for dropping the ball.

It is almost axiomatic that as you have just the one prostate, you have only one shot at getting it right, so you and your doctor, surgeon, urologist, oncologist need to give some very careful thought to how you should progress and should consider all the options.

Nothing too revolutionary so far; however, the following is my comment for today. In trying to learn a bit more about what is happening to me, I've been using myself as a case study, reading a few books, talking to a few fellow sufferers and various medicos and checking out the Net. Now, we all know the Internet can throw up anything from graffiti on the lavatory wall to great insight and many points in between, but there appear to be a large number of prostate specialists, particularly in the States, who have set up treatment centres that specifically evangelise for one treatment over another. They might be right, they might not be, but one thing is for sure: they have a big expense base and need revenue. Old sick men with a few grey dollars may not be too difficult a market. Crumbs! Maybe I'm getting too cynical. Perhaps I should have gone rowing today.

Thursday, 17 November 2005

I'm sitting on the 11.44 from Lingfield station, daydreaming out of the window. It's a clear, sunny day; there was a hard frost overnight and we didn't put the agapanthus inside. It's warm inside the train, and, since you ask, it's £9.60 return. Maybe the car has had its day. In the new rolling stock, we glide past fields I have never been to, but know so well.

Earlier this morning, I went on the erg. I did a 19-minute pyramid, starting with 2 easy minutes, then 1, 2, 3, 2, 1 minutes of hard work, each sandwiched between 2 minutes of easy going.

Before 5 June 2005, I'd hold a rate of about 1 min. 37 sec. for 500 m for each of the work pieces; now, for what seems to be a similar level of effort, it's about 1 min. 44 sec. It's impossible to be precise, but it is about a 5 per cent loss in physical performance. This is another place from where I was. This, to me, has been the most noticeable side effect of the hormone therapy. Dr Sneddon had been right. 'You do realise that taking these hormone tablets, when this is all over, will probably impact your 2,000-m indoor-rowing times.'

I know I am repeating myself, but as with the PSA number, it's the change and more specifically the rate of change that is the important dynamic variable, and, for me, there is no better ruler or measurement than the erg scores.

I feel no symptoms from the cancer; there is still an awareness in my right shoulder, particularly first thing in the morning, but I've decided there are no sharks in Kalamata Bay, and even if there are, they should be preserved and not feared. The only side effect of cancer to date is that I value life and know I am loved.

Two nil. I win. Maybe. Or is this just the half-time score?

The possibility of another pulmonary embolism is held at bay by the warfarin, and the only side effects of it are that I get to chat with Lynne and that (possibly with the help of my own body's defence system) the varicose veins in my calf and the big hard black vein I had on my upper thigh seem to have disappeared.

So that just leaves the side effects of the monthly Zoladex shot. Long term, the bouncy prof was talking about diabetes and bone thinning being on the agenda to join the short-term effects. I may, at some time, be concerned about the long term, but right now, the future being guaranteed to no one, particularly me, I'll just consider the short-term effects. I think, after nearly five months of this stuff, I have been fortunate.

Jonathan, the sailor with dreams that will be realised in five days' time when the ARC fleet leaves Las Palmas, picked up a liver problem almost immediately after starting the hormone treatment. George, the guy who works in the gardening centre, is still getting hot flushes two years after stopping three years' worth of hormone treatment and radiotherapy. To date, I've been spared both these symptoms.

Added to which, I still seem to get erections and to be able to ejaculate, although I have almost no interest in sex. I certainly don't need to shave every day any more, but do so out of habit. I do seem to have lost body hair, and if anything, the hair on my head is thicker. I weigh around 115 kg, which is the same weight I was before my hospital stay. My shape has changed marginally, but I still get into my trousers, and I don't think I'm developing breasts. My testicles in particular and my penis did seem to shrink in August, but I've either got used to them or they too are the same size as before 5 June, OK but modest. (Actually, I've just read that eight out of ten men are not happy with their penile length. What I want to know is, all my life, why do those two out of ten always stand by me in the showers?)

So that just leaves the drugs impacting my erg scores. This is not so apparent in actual rowing. Rak and I won our veteran pairs race a few weeks ago, and last Sunday I competed in a pick-up crew in a coxless four in the Fours Head. We were rowing up a veteran grade and we still came third. In fact, if I competed in the British Indoor Rowing Championships this Sunday, 20 November, even with a 5 per cent drug deficit, I might still have won. Exercise may be good for many reasons, but at the moment perhaps it's better not to put myself on the line. I wasn't prepared to turn up just to compete, not yet, anyway.

As I have already mentioned, I am a walking pharmacy at the moment. I'm just going to have to adjust to the 5 per cent drug-deficit tariff that has to be paid. Here I am with locally advanced prostate cancer, beyond surgery, and in December maybe I'll be told there is no point in radiotherapy, and I'm worrying about a 5 per cent reduction in my athletic performance at the age of 57. Grow up and count your blessings. Yeah, but if I do have radiotherapy and it works and I keep on taking the Zoladex for three years like I told the bouncy prof I would as part of his experiment, maybe that 5 per cent deficit will just fall away with no effort.

Hurst Green, five minutes down the line. I stop staring vaguely out of the window at the sun-dappled mosaic of rural Surrey, pony paddock land, and pick up the book I'm nursing. I've been sent five copies of *It's Not About the Bike*, and now I've been sent a copy of *L.A. Confidentiel: Les secrets de Lance Armstrong*, published in 2004, and it's in French. Hey, look at me, aren't I the king kiddie? I'm reading a book in French.

Mr Sidney G.F. Lawes was my first form master and French *teacher*. In 1959, at the age of eleven, thirty of us in our brand new big blazers, bought large enough for us to grow into for at least two years, stood in front of him on our first day at Greenway Comprehensive School for Boys, Southmead, Bristol. He had an ulcer from the war and he loved France; he didn't love us, but he wanted us to love all things French. So, a couple of years on, I found myself on a one-month school exchange programme, living with Philippe Delas and his family at 57 Rue Tranchère, Bordeaux. When Philippe came to stay with me, he fell in love with my sister Eileen – everyone did. I am loving writing this! For me, Cesare Pavese got it more or less right when he said, 'The richness of life lies in the memories we have forgotten.' Maybe, if Cesare allows me, I could just put in the word 'almost' ahead of 'forgotten'. We're still at Hurst Green.

Roll on a few years from Greenway Comprehensive to early 1973. I'm sitting in the Hilton Hotel at the black-tie dinner following the England v. France match (we actually won), next to Christopher Wayne Ralston. Wayne is really big, a couple of years older than me but light years ahead of me in life. He's original, he likes cigars (really he likes cigarettes, but currently he's in training) and nightclubs, he is the Kings Road personified, a habitué of the famous Queen's Elm pub, and Marie Ange is his French wife. Chris has played for Paris Université Club (PUC, pronounced 'puke' – I like that). After the meal and speeches, a well-built (OK, fat), black-tied, swarthy, richly crumpled, warm, round-faced man shambles up to Chris and says hello. Chris stands up to shake his hand; Chris doesn't usually stand up, what with his bad knee, to shake people's hands.

It is Gérard Krotoff, president of PUC. Chris introduces us.

You know how sometimes you like people for no reason? Well, I liked Gérard. He liked me and he liked life. In part, he liked me because, as a younger man, he had played at Harlequins RFC, and he had fond Anglophile leanings. He was that unusual Frenchman who actually likes the English, and he knew a song about Polly Perkins from Paddington Green. Within a few minutes, he'd asked me if next season I'd like to play for PUC for a while. I say, 'Why not?' and that I'll be there in mid-September.

At the time I was at the LSE, and England were due to travel to Argentina in May, and I'd fixed up a job with Midland Bank to start in September. I phoned the bank up, and they said a January start was fine, and Peter Berryman, the coach at Rosslyn Park, said, 'Good idea.' Oh, those lovely forgotten violent amateur days!

I then did something that even now I feel ashamed about. It was the action of a weak, selfish, thoughtless man. All that year of 1972–3, I had lived with Moya in a house with five girls and another guy in Chelsea. Crumbs, we had it easy! A student on a grant and a scholarship living just off the smart end of the Kings Road, and you could park your car, or in my case bike, outside for no charge. Moya was great and so were her family, who all that year only ever showed me love and kindness. I think she wanted to make the relationship more permanent, but it wasn't the right time for me. Instead of sitting down with Moya and telling her just that, which would have been difficult but the best thing to have done (I mean, that's sort of what Sally Jones did to me when she dumped me after we finished at UEA), this is what I did. I wrote a letter, left it on a table in her flat, got on my bike and ran off to Paris. What a complete shit. And here is the really bad bit: sitting on my bike on the A16 out of Calais, I didn't give Moya a second thought. I have since.

It was a warm late-September evening when I got to Paris. All I knew was that PUC played at Stade Charléty. I found the stadium. There was a bar and it was open. With the PUC, there was always a bar and it was always open. Shit that I was, I had fallen amongst angels.

Gérard was surprised to see me. I couldn't help but love him, although actually it should have been quite easy to dislike him: he was prejudiced, dictatorial and capricious. He liked me in part because I was a 'star', and he allowed me a latitude he gave to no one else in the team. The boys must have really loved me for that. The left-wing revolutionary element of the club (and even in the PUC, a bastion of the old order, there is always going to be a left-wing revolutionary element – this was France *circa* 1973 after all) also sort of loved Gérard, but in a left-wing revolutionary sort of way.

So whenever and wherever he stood up, the cry 'Krotoff – Pinochet!' would echo around him, and as his obvious displeasure grew exponentially, everyone would join in the cry. He was French, he would get very emotional. Normally, I don't like dictators, but Gérard only really genuinely hated one group, and that was the Racing Club de Paris rugby team. In that hatred, we, as members of PUC, were happy to give him our full support. I never found out why he, and consequently we, despised Racing Club de Paris, but then hatred is an emotion and not a rational feeling.

Gérard's petite and charming wife, Josette, who came from the Haute-Savoie and had competed in the 1964 Winter Olympics at Innsbruck, loved Paris and acted as my escort to a city that I also, like many before me, have loved ever since. In between life, to earn some money, I was *l'entraîneur* for the rugby team at the Grande École Polytechnique. I was only in Paris for three months; it seemed, in the nicest way, much longer. The following year, I went on tour with PUC to New Zealand, visiting LA and some of the old French possessions, New Caledonia and Tahiti.

In fact – and I still think this must be some sort of record – we played a match on a Saturday in Auckland, took a plane that evening and flew to Tahiti, crossing the International Date Line, and then played another team in Tahiti on the same Saturday afternoon. I do remember we lost both games. The real high spot of this tour, however, was not this carelessness of losing twice in one day in two different islands about 5,000 miles from each other, or the number of times the entire touring party was naked (like everywhere, anywhere), but the match in the Valley in Los Angeles. Rugby in the USA is a cult thing, played largely in colleges or by teams of older guys. PUC could be quite brutal for no apparent reason, and in this match, they were at their worst. The Americans put up with it for a while and then decided this was their chance to rerun the Alamo. The match was abandoned in acrimony, blood and confusion.

Both sides met afterwards in some big poolside house. I think it was some French ambassadorial place, because the entire touring team were in their very best attire. The Americans didn't speak French and weren't happy and were looking like, well, like angry Californians. The French, who spoke little English, had moved on emotionally from the game and just couldn't understand why the Americans weren't happy. The young PUC captain asked me why; I explained that the Californians thought we were a bunch of privileged French jerks. He immediately lined the team up, and in single file, fully attired, glasses in hand, we said sorry and walked into the pool. In so doing, actually confirming that we were a bunch of privileged French jerks. However, the Americans appreciated the gesture, so they also jumped in, and everyone got cut feet and wasted. Actually, you had to be there, but the entente was more than patched up. Gérard was beaming and very wet.

Josette died young of cancer in the late 1970s, and then, about 20 years later, Gérard got the same disease. The last time I saw him, I rowed (105 hours) from London to Paris. Two teams of seven in a fixed-seat pilot cutter, three hours on, three hours off, start at Big Ben, right at Ramsgate, round to Dover, across the channel and up the Seine to the Eiffel Tower.

We met in one of those big fancy hotels off the Place de la Concorde. We found a quiet lounge there with a big open fire. It was mid-morning, and except, bizarrely, for a harpist, it was empty. He had made a huge effort to get there; he looked smart, thin and poorly, but seemed delighted that I had rowed there, as he said, just to see him. Which I had. I waved goodbye outside the hotel as he went off in a taxi; he waved back. I never saw him again. It was two years before he died. Cancer can squeeze long and hard.

I went to his funeral with John Hall, a good friend. The church, about 30 miles west of Paris, was packed with big men with broken faces, limping because of worn-out knees, hips and ankles. The service was taken by a curious priest who had a tape recorder. I've never understood France.

Platform six, East Croydon station, over to platform two and pick up the Brighton-to-Bedford Thameslink, first stop London Bridge. I start to read the book, in French. Just a few pages in, and I'm wondering how did Lance upset these guys, this isn't *It's Not About the Bike*. The book really seemed to have it in for him. I still don't understand why there is a 'get Lance Armstrong' industry; still, I'll read the book and maybe find out.

Armstrong seems to be viewed differently by the French, and the difference, in part, is like the title of that film, *Lost in Translation*. (Personally, I wanted to shake the two spoilt characters and suggest they should do something to get over their ennui. Like how about reading a book?) In English, the title of Lance's autobiography, *It's Not About the Bike*, almost begs the question, 'Well, what is it about?' The answer is, of course, it's about fighting through the adversity of a less than silver-spooned upbringing and the ravages of cancer to overcome all obstacles and win what is perhaps the greatest sporting endurance test in the world not once but seven times. Heroic. (Although I suppose, if you wanted to take a more world-weary cynical view, you might say the answer to the question is, 'It's not about the bike, it's about the money.') However, in France, Lance's book is translated as *Il n'y a pas que le vélo dans la vie*. 'There is more to life than cycling.' Or maybe, 'In life, there are other things than the bike.' Either way, this is more of a simple statement than the Anglo-Saxon, fighting, inspirational title, which demands some sort of response. This got lost in translation.

The train pulls into London Bridge. I'm going to a City rugby lunch in the Bengal Clipper, an Esher Rugby Club fundraiser organised by Hugh McHardy, then the Esher coach. It's brilliant. I continue to be blown away by the kindness of everyone, particularly those in the rugby world. But I'm kinda worried. Working on the basis that people have an attention span somewhere between that of a gnat and an absolute top whack of three months, where's that going to leave me when the spotlight moves on, a few weeks down the road?

Saturday, 19 November 2005

You know the early-morning deal, as of course do I, having lived it for the last ten years. Blinking orange light, 6.30, toast, Torben, Tideway Scullers at Chiswick. It's now high-pressure winter weather: hard frost during the night, no wind and sunny days; soon we will need lights on the boat at 7.30, but not yet. Christmas and Midwinter's Day are still five weeks away. We go out in a coxless four, which in my case is very appropriate. Cold, frosty, flat almost still water gently ebbing, fog lifting, the rattle of the Tube train going over the Victorian iron-girdered Kew Railway Bridge, blades in the water, leaving it out there. It's magical. Shower, quick cup of tea, then over to Sky TV at Osterley.

Today, England are playing the All Blacks at Twickenham, but I'm not going there for that. Nope, since Paul's *Sunday Times* report, some people have got my phone number and I'm now rent-a-gob. I'm going to be one of the contributors to a 15-minute report on prostate cancer for Channel 501. The other contributors are Professor Roger Kirby, the prostate-cancer specialist, who recently helped set up a prostate disease charity and a clinic in Wimpole Street, and Dr Chris Hiley, who is the head of policy and research at The Prostate Cancer Charity. Within one second of meeting her, you know she is an able, gentle woman. Kate Stewart, head of media and public affairs for the same charity, kindly also came along to see we were all comfortable.

I get to the Sky studios early; Roger is sitting alone in the green room. Now, normally, when a man with prostate cancer meets Roger, the relationship is self-evident. He is the man who is going to cut you up. He is the man who is going to give you the news, one way or the other; he is the man who is going to save your life or not, or improve your quality of life or not. He is unequivocally the man. As with Mike Swinn on 24 June 2005 at East Surrey Hospital, I feel a wave of sympathy. What a burden to carry. Roger looked fine but quite careworn; no wonder, with so many people's lives literally in his hands – or maybe he'd just had a late night.

There was one crucial difference between today and 24 June, and that was that I now know, as important as Mike and Roger are, that I'm part of the system, I have my own bespoke cancer and my future lies more in my hands than those of anybody else. I feel respectful and sympathetic to the surgeons, but not necessarily deferential. I have reclaimed the responsibility for my life. The burden, or joy, is mine, and I own it and I can do what I like with it. Comfortingly, I also know that if it is within their powers, they will help me. But the cancer belongs to me. It will not be outsourced. It is mine.

Roger and I talk as equals, fellow panellists. He asks, I reply. I know the script: PSA 133, Gleason 7, hormone therapy, locally advanced, MRI scan, probable local spread/possible metastatic spread, bone scan clear, being treated by the prof and the doc at the Marsden, PSA fell monthly – 95, 3.2, 1.1 – next test 14 December and maybe a decision then as to whether radiotherapy will be worthwhile and the possibility of a cure (which also depends on the availability of current NHS resources), or maybe just a limited extension of a piece of string. Roger says I'll make 60.

The support of my family and friends and particularly the rugby world has given me a surprising strength. I can bore for Britain and talk quite openly about anything: erectile dysfunction, my erectile dysfunction, incontinence, death, rectal examinations, shrinking testicles, penile size, whatever. For me, at present, there is no taboo subject. I am enjoying this.

Other than the obvious criticisms of vanity, ego, etc., I do have one further concern about going on TV to recommend that men get checked to find out if they have prostate cancer. May I first cover this with a million caveats, all based around the fact that just having prostate cancer doesn't make you an expert. It may make you more interesting on a TV panel, since death is on your shoulder and death row has always had a macabre fascination for the living, but please understand I actually know little. I've also got to throw this in as well, because I believe this is the line of The Prostate Cancer Charity, for whom I have only the highest regard: the earlier you find out about cancer, the more likely it is you can treat it, so if you are at risk, get a DRE and then if necessary a PSA test and then if necessary have a biopsy and then if necessary a radical prostatectomy or radiotherapy or hormone treatment. I am on message here, but it is probably the right message.

However, consider this: 'It is believed that up to 80% of all men develop prostate cancer by the age of 80. Nothing like this number of men suffer harm from their cancer, implying that in most men prostate cancer is a harmless illness.' (*Prostate Cancer: The Facts*, M. Mason and L. Moffat)

Now, M. Mason and L. Moffat, try telling that to the one person who dies of prostate cancer each hour of each day of each week of each month of each year. However, the two viewpoints are reconcilable.

We know cancers, for practical reasons, are defined by where they originate in the body. We know each cancer is bespoke to the individual and will have its own characteristics, its own identity. Each rogue cell has its own potential characteristics and structure and growth pattern. Maybe the cancer, when contained in the prostate, is harmless, and only when it spreads out of the prostate will it grow rapidly, act like many other cancers and perhaps metastasise. What men die of is not cancer in the prostate but cancer in the prostate that has the characteristics to grow out of the prostate and become, say, bone cancer.

This gives rise to further doubts and questions but I will try to address only two here. First, why does cancer in the prostate appear to move so slowly when it is contained in the prostate? Well, actually, does it? The answer would seem to be yes. Although cancer even in the prostate will move according to its individual characteristics – all cancers will change and move at different speeds – maybe, just maybe, there is something in the prostate which limits, delays, defers the growth and spread of certain cancers while they are contained in the prostate. If the cancer is not likely to spread out of the prostate and there are no urinary problems, why not just leave it alone? Why have all the additional complications of the slash, fry and poison treatment when there may be no need? There is at present no method of identifying the cancers that will spread, so all cancers in men of a certain age will tend to be treated, unless there are resource shortages.

Second, there are definitional issues when it comes to describing your cancer in a way that tells you more about it than simply its place of origin. The definition of your cancer – how aggressive it is, how quickly it is likely to advance – is usually based around the Gleason score. The Gleason test can be tremendously useful, but it is more than 40 years old, and it can also be flawed, depending as it does on the samples taken during the biopsy and on the pathologist's interpretation of these. There is no test that is universally accepted as being able to define for you the true nature of your cancer, which means that choosing the correct treatment is in some cases a matter of guesswork – informed, skilled guesswork but guesswork nonetheless.

We have missed our slot at 10.45 because of some breaking news. Kate Stewart shows her teeth and we have our say a half-hour later. We all push the awareness theme and stress that a DRE is something that is very worthwhile, which of course it is. Sure, there is a bit of a dignity hurdle to jump, but a DRE may save your life, and at the very least, it will put your mind at rest. Roger rushed off afterwards to do good works. God be with you, Roger.

Whereas I rushed off to an easier option: lunch at Rosslyn Park before watching them play Dings Crusaders. Although before I left Sky, I was asked to sit on another panel, to give my view on the England–All Blacks match later that afternoon. Funny old life. From the same seat, one minute you're advising people to let their doctor make a rectal examination and the next you're discussing the shoving technique of the England loose-head and hooker. Life's a lark.

Wednesday, 23 November 2005

'He's a man way out there in the blue, riding on a smile and a shoeshine . . . a prostate-cancer sufferer has got to dream, boy.' (With apologies, obviously, to Arthur Miller.) Or maybe, as Henry David Thoreau wrote, 'Dreams are the touchstones of our characters.' And maybe, as I wallow in nostalgia, reside in Amnesia Avenue and slip down any old sentimental side street in a storm, I can even find myself disagreeing with Thomas Jefferson, because today he's dead and today I'm not, when he writes, 'I like the dreams of the future better than the history of the past.'

Sure, Tom, dreams are great, but I had intended today to wallow in the history of the past and think about exercise and how, on our wonderful family summer holidays in Crantock, Cornwall, in the 1950s, by competing in the church-organised summer fete foot-races for under-fives, I discovered I could run and how ever since I have been seduced by sport and exercise and how it has enriched my life.

Nah, I'll let that sit for another day. Dreams are great as well as history, but right now, the best is hope.

I haven't written for a few days because I felt I could do better than when I wrote last, four days ago, and left dangling, just dangling, so many doubts and uncertainties. I must do better. Not only for myself but for other prostate-cancer sufferers who may read this. Great as they are, unthreaded dreams are not enough. *The Field of Dreams* may have been a great film, but what we prostate-cancer sufferers need is the field of hope, which is not the same place. First hope, then dreams. Hope is the hors d'oeuvre to the dreams of life.

There is hope. Treatment has improved beyond measure; if you're gonna get cancer get it in the twenty-first century. There is hope. Diagnosis and testing for cancer has improved beyond measure.

But what is actually being treated? What is actually being diagnosed? Each cancer has its own character, which is unknown and can only be guessed at – an informed guess made by an experienced pathologist with a microscope, but still a guess. C'mon, Dr Gleason of the twenty-first century, you just gotta be out there somewhere. Pick up the torch, turn the dream into hope and hope into reality for all us old men hanging on the wire, being brave. Help us.

Now, in early-stage cancer, for example, will treatment be given, with the attendant side effects, when maybe that cancer would never have grown or caused damage? You might be cured, but perhaps you were never under threat, and now you are winged in some way. On the other hand, perhaps because of the characteristics of that early-stage cancer, even all the king's horses and all the king's men would not have been able to prevent its growth.

Am I saying treatment in the early stages is a waste of time because it may harm you, it cannot be undone and it is the unknown characteristics of your cancer that will dictate how events unfurl?

No. I think what I am saying is take control, understand what is happening to you, consider the options, own your cancer. Nobody knows you as well as yourself. Listen and trust your doctors, but it's your disease, not theirs. Then live your life, love your life.

So, sage of Dormansland, man with the big brave gob, what are you going to do now?

Listen to the doctor, take the hormone injections, with all the actual and possible Faustian-pact add-ons. If the next visit to the Marsden on 14 December shows a rise in my PSA, then it probably means that life will be less long than I would have wished and there is probably little point in radiotherapy, of whatever variety, and then I'll follow my own advice and make sure I enjoy whatever remains. If the PSA has stayed low and the opportunity of radiotherapy is there, I'll take it with both hands, in the full knowledge of the possible consequences of the potential side effects. In any event, it'll be my call, with my eyes wide open.

In the meantime, I'll live each day, and tomorrow I'll wallow back into the joy of my life and Crantock and exercise. Goodnight. Sweet dreams.

Thursday, 24 November 2005

Today is exactly five months on to the day when Mike had the conversation with me. When Elisabeth and me and Tim and Maria had been lolling about on a patch of what might one day be grass, under two big oak trees, through the door marked 'Strictly No Exit', and we were waiting, just waiting in the sunshine, and it was a wonderful warm day. You remember.

Well, today it's five months on, and I'm feeling extremely perky. I had intended carrying on in the same sort of vein as yesterday, about taking ownership and so on, and helping yourself by considering diet and particularly exercise; I'd planned to revisit 1952 and Crantock. Well, maybe I will, but others have done this, especially about diet, much better; and eventually I may get on my marks at Crantock, but something else has just cropped up.

Now this could be the drugs kicking in or maybe I'm just going nuts, but today I know my cancer is female. I think earlier on I mentioned I was having an affair with my illness; well I am. I'm just hoping Elisabeth doesn't find out.

So far, actually from the very beginning, some five months ago, she hasn't been too demanding, although quite frankly she was not my choice, and she knows that. In fact, I've been trying to get rid of her almost from the very start, to poison her actually, which has created a few problems for me and her, but none, hopefully, that I can't handle.

Really, I should have just cut her out from the start, but women, they are so gorgeous, and she'd got too big a hold on me. So cutting her dead, well, it wouldn't have worked. I suppose her coming to live with me was a big mistake, but it wasn't my choice. She just moved in without even asking me, baggage and all, which she is threatening to spread over the whole house. If it had been her place, true to form, I could just have written a letter, jumped on my bike and headed on down the A16 from Calais without a second thought. This time, difficult as it may be, we are going to have to have a little chat.

Though it's not all bad, her living with me. Everyone is really sympathetic. They know she wants me all to herself, but she can't have that and never will. Sure, maybe she can have my body, but she'll never have my heart. Never, ever. I'd sooner die first.

OK, on your marks, get set, go, Crantock . . . Another false start. Next time I'll be disqualified.

I've got to add on that last night I went to the Lloyd's of London rugby club dinner as a guest of Ralph Sharpe, whom I'd worked with on some board or other at Lloyd's. Ralph is the current chairman of the rugby club, and he has always been kind to me. Anyway, being the chairman, he introduced the guest speaker, David Trick. Tricky was a speedy winger for Bath and England in the 1980s (as my career was ending, his was beginning), and he has learned how to do after-dinner speaking. He's self-deprecating, funny and entertaining, and it's a good way of earning your livelihood. Tricky knows the script, and I've always liked him.

There is a bond with people you've played with and against. Those who played before you were rubbish, and those who came after you are also, obviously, rubbish. No, that bond exists, and exists forever, only with those who served with you and against you at the same time in the trenches. They are special. So David Trick, to me, is special, as I hope I am to him. Ralph, possibly because the club was paying for the speaker, introduced Tricky in a sort of deprecating, off-hand employer–employee manner. Now, whereas Tricky can do self-deprecation, he ain't going to take it from anyone else, except maybe his fellow trenchees. There is a bit of a golden rule in after-dinner speaking, and that is never, ever diss the person who is going to speak after you. Ralph didn't pay heed to this golden rule. We all laughed, although I think, during the next 20 minutes or so, Ralph learned the true meaning of the expression 'through gritted teeth'.

I was aware of three other things last night. First, in late November when it's cold and wet and late and you've been poorly, wearing a coat is a really, really good idea. Second, I've often spoken at dinners (c'mon, babes, give the spotlight to me, dontcha know I, the self-publicist, need it), but now I feel I genuinely have no need for that. I now know who I am, I'm happy with the way things are. My insecurity, if that's what it was, no longer needs feeding. It's OK because *she*'s with me. Finally, as ever, I am still just blown away by the concern people, many of whom I hardly ever knew, seem to have for me. It is humbling and I love it.

Saturday, 26 November 2005

Diet. If you diet drastically, you'll diet many times, because your weight loss will last only for a short while, until the cry of the uneaten Hob Nobs becomes louder than your ever-diminishing willpower. If you want to lose weight and make it permanent, there's more to it than binge starving or dehydrating yourself. A permanent but not too dramatic change in lifestyle is required, which should include exercising as well as watching what you eat and drink.

Diet is self-evidently not just about weight; is has a lot to do with well-being, nutrition and health. We all want to look and feel good about ourselves until we die, and we probably want that to be later than sooner. So vanity and mortality are the unequal drivers of healthy eating.

I've never dieted, because I've been an exercise junkie all my life. A side benefit of that obsession is that I have been able to eat what I like, and I do, and I always have done so. As a consequence of that exercise obsession, my concerns about mortality and vanity were indirectly addressed. Until recently, I had the same shape as 30 years ago. I exercise, eat relatively healthily, drink in moderation and have never smoked, so I believed that the only threat to my life I had to worry about was an accident, that death wasn't, for me, a health issue. Got that completely wrong, Andrew.

I love eating, and since 24 June, I have still made no concessions to what or how much I eat. In fact, right now, I'm eating even more, because *she* has made me really popular. People are so kind. Last night I went out to Lead Yacht's directors' Christmas dinner with Peter Sangster, the chairman, Linda, his wife of one year, Allan, who underwrites the business, his wife, Cheryl, Vlad and his wife, Lucy. It's a great meal. We have it in the Cavalry and Guards Club at 127 Piccadilly, and there is a regimental reunion dinner filling the place with noise and joy.

What do I eat? Lobster bisque and lots of bread, two glasses of Pouilly Fumé, a huge rib-eye steak with all the trimmings and three glasses of a heavy red, profiteroles, cheese, coffee and a very nice dessert glass of Sauternes. Should I be eating this? Well, why not? Perhaps because I had a not dissimilar meal the evening before, and our friend Jane Surtees has kindly invited Elisabeth and myself to her 50th birthday dinner this evening, and as Christmas approaches, so does the gourmet pace step up.

All this eating means that I'm facing three issues. First, the hormone treatment can result in the patient putting on 15 to 20 lb, usually around the waist. Although I still weigh about 115 kg, my shape is changing. For the first time, I cannot get into my 36-in.-waist trousers and 38-in. waistbands are beginning to be a bit of a challenge. All my clothes, suits, jeans – none have a waist of more than 38 in. I am now wearing my T-shirts over my trousers and not tucking them in, and I suddenly recognise that black can hide a lot. I am also developing an embryonic belly, which I've never had to worry about before. But the worst thing is the roll of fat on my pubic bone. I know what the answer is, but can I eat less?

The second issue is that there is also a health aspect to this. Most of the books I've bought say there may be a strong correlation between prostate cancer and dairy products and saturated fats. It's possible that food-wise I'm doing the equivalent of smoking 40 a day. I am not eating fried tomato skins or taking selenium supplements or doing any of the other good and sensible things one is recommended to do.

The third issue is that although my appetite for food, probably seasonally adjusted, is at least the same as ever, my appetite for exercise seems to be diminishing. Today is the first Saturday morning in a long time I have not gone rowing. It's cold, I had a late night, etc., etc. Also, my interest in sitting on the ergometer seems to be diminishing. It seems such an effort to do what I once did so easily. Torben may be my saviour; he forces me to take him for a long walk every day. Again, as with the food concern, I know what the answer is: just get on with it. But can I? It's not too difficult, I know that just doing it is more important than really doing it.

Perhaps those two drivers, vanity and mortality, aren't

kicking in any more? No. I am as vain as ever, albeit with little foundation. I really don't like what is starting to happen to me physically, but if I'm that bothered, I'll do something about it. It's the second driver that is a problem: mortality. If I find out on 14 December that my PSA has risen, why bother? If my future is only a piece of string, why bother doing anything? Why not, after 57 years, just let myself go? Are there any prizes for having the thinnest corpse in the cemetery? Is this giving up? Maybe I'm on the edge here. I can't control much, but I can control what I put in my mouth and what exercise I take. I'll come back to all this.

Besides the diet and exercise concerns, I also seem to be changing within myself. The hormone injections are doing things to me physically, none of them too bad, no immediate liver damage or hot flushes. In fact, the side effects are almost beneficial, fat on the pubic bone and a loss of libido apart. I wrote in my third email, of 14 July: 'Side effects while taking the drug: impotence and muscle loss, possible hot flushes and generally getting in touch with your feminine side. Can't wait.'

Can't wait. Well, I was right – and lucky. I have got in touch with my feminine side, and it is great. I was a fantastic human being before but now, now, I am just really brilliant. It may be that people seem to be being kind to me and asking me out more than ever before because they feel sorry for me or they want to let me know that they're with me, standing by me when times are tough. These may be the reasons, but I think it is because I am now a truly brilliant bloke, and they just want to be in my fantastic company because I'm so great. Why am I so great? I'll tell you. Because for the first time in my life, I listen to what people tell me rather than talking to them about me. Everybody has their own story, everybody has their own secrets, their own issues, their own concerns, their own stuff. And do you know what? Theirs are probably more interesting than yours, or, in my case, mine.

For example, at the dinner at 127 Piccadilly, because I listened, I found out that Vlad's granddad was the Serbian ambassador to the Vatican at the beginning of the Second World War and that his son, Vlad's dad, used to nick the diplomatic car to go visiting brothels in Rome. I heard that Allan had just been on a stag night in Prague and that at two in the morning in a McDonald's he had witnessed the best man in the kids' ball pool meeting a Czech lady. As he said, two cultures had collided; I didn't ask him what that meant. I discovered that Peter had met his new wife (both were recently bereaved) through an Internet site and had proposed to her within 13 days and that, against all expectations, he and Linda were really happy.

I really should take every opportunity to keep my mouth shut and listen. If people know she is inside, you don't have to tell them, they know. It's easy. Just do what women have been doing since time began: be a pair of ears and simply listen. That'll keep those invites flowing. Eat well but less, move about, it'll be fine. And never stay down. I'm no longer on the edge; life is too brilliant not to give it your best shot forever.

Sunday, 27 November 2005

First Sunday of Advent. The candle for the patriarchs – Abraham, Joshua and Isaac – is lit. Georgie Best died on Friday, one of Peter Pan's lost boys.

Monday, 28 November 2005

'Life is too brilliant not to give it your best shot forever.' I suppose this is almost an aphorism, but whatever it is, it turns on the individual's definition of 'best shot'.

At East Surrey Hospital, when a group of guys huddled together in the cold outside the building to smoke, I suppose they were, in a sense, giving it their best shot. Personally, I've never smoked and think it is a nasty little habit. However, there is also something perhaps even romantic about people knowing the dangers and nonetheless exercising their right to do something that is not good for them. Although, actually, the cardio ward at East Surrey was many things, but romantic probably wasn't one of them.

I suppose there are many types of obsession – smoking, eating, drinking, money, sex, power – and if you could just harm yourself and nobody else, then what would be wrong with having one? But that's almost never possible; obsessions tend to corrode, physically or emotionally, everything around them. 'It's my little treat.' Yeah, right.

My obsession has always been exercise, but maybe that's a rare benign obsession. Maybe. So 'best shot' for me includes many things, and exercise is big in the mix. But since I've been taking both the daily dose of warfarin and the 28-day hormone injection, my fitness level, as indicated by my performance on the rowing ergometer, has fallen by about 5 per cent and so too has my enthusiasm for exercise. The two may be connected.

I still don't know what will happen on 14 December, on my third visit to the Marsden. On both my two previous visits, I had been hoping to be offered some certainty; now I know this was an unrealistic hope. Good guys that the white coats are, they don't know what the future holds. They will take their cue from the PSA test result.

I have decided not to try to pre-empt what may or may not happen following the 14 December meeting, but my hope is that my PSA has stayed down, that in January I'll be put on a six-week course of radiotherapy, that the Prof will let me off the hormone treatment after, say, another year, that I'll be taken off the warfarin, and so by this time next year, I'll be in training for the 60–65 age group at the World Indoor Rowing Championships. That's what I'm hoping. But in the meantime, I'll write about what I'm doing now.

That old adage 'The past is history, the future is a mystery and today is a gift' is, like most old adages, not wrong. I'll keep my hopes for the future in my head, but now I'd like to go back to the start of my exercise obsession – Crantock – and then up to the gift of today. (For those with cancer, this stuff on exercise may or may not be useful, because we all start from different places and are at different stages, and, as you know, this is selfishly about me.)

I think there is little downside in physical activity. The benefits are not only those of potentially improving your physical condition and, in spite of everything, trying to maintain a healthy body weight; the best part is often in your head.

Does it matter what sort of exercise you do? I don't think so. Just moving your body, or those parts of it that you can, in some sort of daily routine is the challenge. For each of us, that challenge will be different. But I'm coming to conclusions before I've even trawled through my history book.

So, at last and eventually and finally, Crantock. Winning the under-fives race, which was a distance of two chains (44 yards) in 1952, was the start of it all. I loved running.

At the age of 13, in 1960, I had a paper round: half a crown a day for the morning round and one shilling and sixpence for the evening one. Most mornings by 6.30 a.m., Mr Pitcher, the newsagent in Coldharbour Road, would already have phoned our house to wake me up, as I hadn't arrived at his shop yet, which drove everyone nuts, particularly Auntie Leah. Sometimes in the morning he'd have to phone me up two or maybe three times, and each time he let the phone ring but not for so long that anyone, specifically Auntie Leah, would actually pick it up.

Then I'd be outside the house, and it was 123 paces from the plane tree in Belvedere Road to the tree at the end of Iddesleigh Road opposite Mr Pitcher's shop. As I grew up, it became my target to run it in under 100 paces, and I think I did. Then I'd run round delivering the papers, except on a Sunday, when they were much heavier. On weekdays I'd go back home, eat breakfast and run to the bus stop on the Downs to catch the 8 or 8A bus to school.

Now, if you've been at that bus stop, you'll know that as the big green double-decker bus comes around the roundabout at the top of Blackboy Hill, you can see only the top of it. It could be an 84 or 84A or a 1 or 1A – completely and utterly useless buses. However, it was my firm belief that if, when you saw the top of the bus, you ran to the white sign which said 'Horse Riders Only On This Side' and got back in time to the bus stop, it would always be an 8 or 8A, and if it wasn't, it was just some dreadful mistake, and it would be OK next time. Inconveniently, as you may well know, it is a request bus stop and not a fare stage, so if you were the only person at the bus stop, you really had to be back in time to put your hand out. I was frequently late for school.

Which was OK, because at Greenway School, in the first
year at least, if you had a blazer and wore a cap and caught
a bus, then you were a fair target for a kicking, which you
would avoid if everyone else was in class by the time you
got there. I loved running, especially away.

Mr Elkins was the sports master and organised the
school cross-country team. Sometimes we could run at
lunchtime, but most of the time we just ran in our PE
lesson (and, of course, away from danger in the school
playground during the breaks). Roger Butterworth and
Nick Hanna, who did not like running, would often sneak
off for a fag during cross country and take a short cut, but
not me, not goody-goody two shoes. Good old Mr Elkins.
He'd take us every year to compete in the Bristol Inter-
Schools Cross Country Championships. I was never really
that good, but I just loved running. I played football in the
winter and did athletics in the summer. The school had a
cinder running track. Greenway was closed down on 20
July 1984; the track was ripped up and the playing fields
sold off, and it is now a community centre.

The school had been an educational experiment. At one
stage, the traditional year classes were abandoned, and
pupils were put into house groups with a range of academic
abilities (huge – most of my group couldn't read). Within
these houses, pupils were divided into groups by ability
and age. You could transfer to a new group at any stage,
which was intended to allow pupils to make the most
of their talents. Strangely, it worked. Why? Because the
brilliant teachers made it work. Eight of us out of a class
of thirty got university grants and scholarships.

In my last year at Greenway, I played a few games of
rugby, but what I really did at school was canoeing. Pixie
Wainwright, the woodwork master, got a group of us,
with our minimum woodworking skill-set, to each build

our own kayak from a kit. It took forever and even longer. We learned to canoe in a local swimming pool, and then, aged 15, one winter Saturday, we went to Builth Wells on the River Wye in Wales, a considerable set of rapids, then and now. With the benefit of hindsight, I suppose we should be grateful no one died; our canoes were trashed. However, a year or two on, enthusiasm untrashed and with the money from the paper round, I'd joined Bristol Canoe Club and bought a second-hand wood-and-canvas Dipper, as well as a 1936 Hillman to transport it with. Magic.

Is it the romantic rose-tinted glasses of an older man looking back on his 18-year-old self or was the post-A-level summer of 1966 just the finest place to be? The generation that had died for us and made our lives possible was discounted, as were their values and culture. The future belonged to us. There was excitement, a social change was happening, and if you were 18, you were at its very centre. The world – for an 18 year old with a place and a grant at the University of East Anglia who had worked on Avonmouth docks all summer and bought a 2.5 litre, fastback, 125 mph 1956 Lancia Aurelia GT with tinted windows, a wood-and-aluminium steering wheel and twin Weber carburettors – was waiting. As was a knackered gearbox halfway up the A11 just north of Thetford. But, hey, man, who needed cars when you could travel by natural velocity?

I've been to three other universities: London School of Economics, Cambridge and a stint at the Sorbonne. None of them even began to compare with UEA in 1966–9. Maybe it was a time and age rather than a place thing. Perhaps nowhere compares to 1966–9. It was a different world, where a boy's worth was measured by the length of his hair: let your freak flag fly. Shallow? You ain't kidding

– but brilliant. Naturally, the world's problems would be solved by music and love. In 1968, I temporarily dropped out at the taxpayer's expense. I followed the very good advice of the Flowerpot Men and went to San Francisco (and all points in between) for five months or so. I picked up the odd job and also the feeling that while 'love and peace' was a great backdrop to my life at the time, maybe it wasn't actually all it was cracked up to be. I obviously wasn't cut out for the hippie lifestyle in the long term: on 4 August 1969, I was to become an articled clerk at Price Waterhouse in the City.

While at UEA, I carried on running. Also, once a week on a Saturday afternoon, Haydn Morris, who had played in the 1955 Lions and was in charge of sport, put me in a rugby shirt, and then, in some muddy field, Norfolk farm-workers would kick the crap out of us in what masqueraded as a game of rugby football.

After university, true heroes went to Goa, or built boats in Norfolk or died. Not me. I went to Rosslyn Park Football Club, where I ran. I ran largely because I liked it and because Sally Jones, with whom I had lived at Wattlefield Hall (a grand old empty house in the middle of Norfolk, in which we'd somehow been lucky enough to end up staying) during the last year of uni, had mercilessly dumped me and broken my heart. And then it was my knee that was broken, playing for Rosslyn Park against Richmond in December '69. Shattered hearts and shattered knees. 1970 could only get better. It did. By the start of the summer, I'd recovered from the injury and had joined the Polytechnic Harriers running club, which was based at the Quintin Hogg sports field in Chiswick.

For the next 20 years, I'm running. In the winter, playing rugby, and I suppose, with a season extending from the last week in August (tour of Cornwall and Devon, not to be missed) to the first week in May (Middlesex Sevens) with an end-of-season tour (usually somewhere hot) and a midweek fixture about every other week, I must have played on average about 55 games a season. I played 20 seasons – so just over 1,000 games for some team or other. Training, injury permitting, was two evening training sessions at the club after work and four long runs at lunchtime during the week. Then we'd play a match Saturday and I'd go for a long easy jog on Sunday.

My final game was on Saturday, 23 April 1989, for Rosslyn Park against Cardiff. I waved farewell a week or so later at the Middlesex Sevens and retired from rugby aged 41.

In the summer, I'd run for Polytechnic Harriers, the high point being in 1978 when I failed to qualify for the 400-m hurdles (with a time of 53.7 sec.) in the Amateur Athletic Association final at Crystal Palace. I'd usually do repetition sprints at West London Stadium four nights a week, plus two weights sessions and two long jogs over four lunchtimes – nothing on Fridays. I loved Fridays. Then I'd compete on Saturday and go for a long steady jog on Sunday. It all seemed quite normal then; I don't know how Elisabeth put up with me.

Athletics gave me up when I was about 37, and so I played for the village cricket team in the summer instead. I bought a bike, joined the East Grinstead Cycling Club as a summer member and competed in the Tuesday-evening 10-mile pursuit. Then I joined the East Grinstead Triathlon Club – swimming two nights a week and lunchtime jogs. A few years on, and Mother Nature began to take her revenge. By my late 40s, she showed no mercy: my knees were shot; I couldn't even jog. No more running for me. Ah well, I'd done enough.

That's when I found rowing, first of all on a machine and then on the water. Splish splosh. I was hooked on this non-weight-bearing activity. For the last ten years or so, I've been rowing maybe three or four mornings a week and on the alternate days going on the ergometer.

All my life, I've never stopped sweating but now it's harder. Is it the cancer? Is it the warfarin? Is it the Zoladex? Is it just me getting old? Or is it something else?

I don't know. I don't really care.

Why not relax?

Because I can't unless I've earned it.

So what am I doing now? At the moment I try to row two mornings a week, on Saturday and Sunday, in a crew boat. It's dark, it's cold, it's 37 miles to Chiswick and I'm poorly, but it has to be done as long as I can do it. Then I try to walk 3 miles a day with the dog 5 times a week and do a 30-minute erg, just to keep my hand in, 3 times a week.

Is this foolish? Maybe, but I want to be active. I want to be alive until I die.

But I'll listen to my body, and then, on 14 December, I'll listen to the doctor. Not that I'll necessarily do what he says. If the news is good, I'll be looking to take that 5 per cent off my ergometer time; if it's bad, well, I'll keep on as long as I can. I've been doing some kind of exercise since I can remember, and I'll carry on that way.

I don't know whether this is good advice to other members of the Cancer Club, but I'd say, bearing in mind you've got to start from where you are, not where you'd like to be, do what you can, and do it on a regular basis.

Thursday, 1 December 2005

There was a time in June when I thought I might not make it, but I have, and today it's my birthday, and I'm 58 and hugely grateful. I have a nice day.

Goethe said there would be little left of him if he were to discard what he owed to others.

Part Two

My intentions were the best. Yesterday, my birthday, seemed like a good and appropriate point to stop writing. I would print out three copies of what I'd written, bind them and give a copy each to Mouse, Clouds and Stef, so they'd know, in spite of everything (and there is always in every life somewhere a bit of everything), that their father and mother loved them.

My reasons for stopping were varied and I thought about them last night, but I can't stop.

She won't let me.

Creepy or what?

Why stop?

First reason: to reclaim my life and live it rather than just observing it.

Second reason: I'd begun to write as if I had some medical knowledge rather than what I'd gleaned from bits and pieces of information, and this might result in bad advice for other members of the Cancer Club, and specifically my branch, the prostate branch. Or even worse, it might make me less sensitive to the real or imagined anxieties and concerns of other sufferers and their families and friends, particularly those who are further down the curve than I am and particularly those in the terminal stage rather than in pre-14 December limbo land. I would hate that. REM. You are not alone. Hang on. Everybody hurts.

Third reason: out of the blue, Price Waterhouse Coopers have phoned me up and asked me to apply to teach a finance course for 80 people. Right up my street: a two-day course in groups of ten, teaching the participants from a base of little or no knowledge how to relate the balance sheet, profit-and-loss account and cash flow to one another, to understand accounting jargon, to keep a set of accounts and, crucially, to not be intimidated by numbers. I can do this, and the potential fee to be earned would make 2006 easy. I should devote my time to convincing those who need to be convinced that I am a good deal and then taking them to PowerPoint heaven. I should spend time working on this, rather than just turning up on 6 December and trying to wing it. Nah, I'll wing it – always have done.

Fourth reason: I was starting to write, without knowing why, random slightly self-indulgent stuff. I was heading towards unveiling my prognostication for the thickening cirrus clouds of concern for the planet in the early part of the twenty-first century, or maybe drifting back to the history of my forebears and the silver cup my great (times five) grandfather won in 1795 in the Skipwith Agricultural Fair in the East Riding of Yorkshire. Nothing wrong with a disconnected stream of consciousness or with self-indulgence if this thing's just for me; but I don't think it is any more.

Fifth reason: following on from that, this account was to be just for me, about me. On 25 August, that's what I'd decided. I'm sure many of us in the Club do and have done the same thing – keeping a diary, keeping a record. It's good therapy and keeping a medical record in particular seems to be a smart idea, part of the process of getting to learn about your cancer, which is pretty important. Learning about your cancer allows you to reach the conclusion that it is yours and that you have to take responsibility, not leave it up to the guys in white coats. Your life may be in their hands, but your cancer is in your body. Own it.

In part, from the start, I also thought, besides helping myself, I'd like to help those in a similar position to that in which I found myself on 24 June when Mr Swinn told me, 'It's unequivocal,' etc. But we all start from different positions, we all have our own bespoke, irregular, differentiated cells doing whatever it is they are doing and will do. We each, individually, have to chart our own course. So, however I dress it up, I can only say how it is for me.

I have reached the end of my road; I have little of further value to say to the Club members, if ever I had anything. I no longer have any need to write for me about me. So that's why yesterday, on my birthday, I decided to stop.

But today I'm still writing.

Am I turning from the sports-mad rugby-playing family-man accountant cancer-sufferer into the double-barrelled Mr Seriously-Weirdo? Is this how it happens?

Who wants me to write? Who am I writing for? Not for me, not for the Club. She wants me to write. I don't know where this is going.

I have been in you now for longer than you care to know. I have never done you harm, Andrew, understand that, and if there has been harm done to you, it is not of my making. Yet you are trying to poison me. Why? Since in the process of weakening me you are weakening yourself, you have lost the edge, the athletic margin, that you have worked for all your life. You have no libido. Although you are not putting on weight, you are getting fatter and losing your shape. None of this is of my making.

Yet you are planning, I know, because you can have no secrets from me, to continue this process of weakening me by burning me and, I might add, in the same process, continuing to harm and weaken yourself. But you know you cannot get rid of all of me, because I am in you. And yet soon you hope to burn out whatever may remain of me and do goodness only knows what damage to yourself in the process. Is this what you really want?

Look, my love, what I have done for you. Since you found out I was in you and with you, have you not had an intensity of life that you had almost forgotten was possible, where every shape and every form and every thought and every emotion is stronger and more life-enhancing than you can ever remember? I have given you this.

Those people who care for you and even those that have never cared for you have become kinder and sweeter and shown you love and emotion and warmth that you might have yearned for but never truly knew was there, and now you know. I have done this for you.

The men and women in white coats whose advice you follow do not care for you like I do. They have their own concerns. To them, you are just a box to be ticked. One way or another. They care even less for me. They don't know me, they just want to slash, fry or poison me. They give me a name, but they don't know me. To them, I am an Escher drawing, stairs rising to a platform lower than themselves, doors leading outside that bring them back inside. They have not tried to untangle me; they treat me as they treat others, but I am different, Andrew, I mean you no harm. We can live together. My love, they wish to turn us into both their meaningful subjects and docile objects. We can live together without them as one.

I cannot let you live. I own you, and forgive me, but if it is within my power, with the help of others, I must kill you.

Monday, 5 December 2005

So last Friday I had a sort of anthropomorphic moment. It's not a her; it's just cancer. I haven't flipped my lid. I'm just scared.

Scared about 14 December. I'll be given the result of my PSA test. I haven't even had the blood test taken yet, but on 14 December, I'll find out if my Perpetual State of Anxiety has bounced up and away, and with it my hopes of radiotherapy, or if it's stayed down and I'll get the chance of a fry 'n' cure. Or maybe some other result.

The good news is I had a great weekend. Two fantastic outings from Chiswick to Richmond on Saturday and Sunday mornings, in a pair and a coxless four. Leaving it out there for Harry. Harry, you would have been proud of me, and I'll make you even prouder. Afterwards on Saturday, I had lunch with Gill and Peter Berryman at Rosslyn Park Rugby Club. Our 1st XV then utterly smashed Hertford RFC 18–10 in a mid-table National League 3 South fixture. Brilliant. Mouse came back from the Dubai Sevens. And Graham, our vicar, based his sermon on this story: a landlord went round collecting rent from his tenants, and at the end of the day he went home and found he had lost from his top inside pocket his wallet with all the takings. He told his wife, who asked him if he'd checked his trousers and the other pockets of his jacket. He said he had done and the wallet wasn't there. His wife then suggested he should look in his overcoat. 'Are you mad?' he said. 'If I looked there – the only place it can now be – and it wasn't there, then I would have no hope left.'

The sermon was about hope, and it struck me that was a pretty convoluted introduction. It was the second Sunday in advent. The candle was lit for the prophets.

If last Friday I had an anthropomorphic moment, then today it's more of a Henry II type moment. Who will rid me of this turbulent disease? But one thing I am sure of, if it ain't good news, then Samuel Johnson's condemned man will eat a hearty breakfast.

If it is a piece of string of indeterminate length, then I will eat metaphorically, 'cause I still wanna look as good as I can and enjoy exercising until, babe, I can exercise and eat no more.

Am I really scared? Yeah. Can I handle it? I think so.

This writing stuff helps and doesn't burden anybody.

'Everybody carries a shadow and the less it is embodied in the individual's conscious life, the blacker and denser it is.' – Carl Jung. Most emotions tend to feed a shadow that obscures the true self. I suppose the shadow is our hidden self, the aspects of our personalities that we don't like to acknowledge or that we have been discouraged from showing. Like, for example, being scared because of what I may be told on 14 December. Are these hidden emotions part of what makes us human? Our shadow side?

My problem, however, is almost the opposite, I have no problem opening up the kimono. In fact, I tend to reveal my shadow side before anyone cares or wants to know. I'm probably the antidote to Freud's ideas about the repressed sides of people. But I believe (for me at least, although this will not apply to all members of the Club) that the longer we persist in disowning the shadow, the darker it becomes. The task of learning to acknowledge our shadows, even to love them and eventually to use their power, is important for me in handling my fear. So today, or now, at least, I can handle it.

For each of us in the Club there is always a date, a point of uncertainty, the next date, the next point, until if we let it, everything becomes pointless because of that date. However, right up until there is finally no date left, there is always a point to life. When my mum was dying, she had lived the last eight years with us in a double garage we had had converted. It was nicer than it sounds. Mum, who was ninety and was always surrounded by love, was three weeks or so in the dying. She was not in too much pain. The guys in white coats (actually, it was the district nurse in her case) can do stuff. Those three weeks gave my siblings, family, in-laws, nephews, nieces and friends time to come to terms with what was happening to Mum and to them and to each other. It was, with the benefit of hindsight, her last and possibly greatest gift to us all: that we should find peace with what was happening and then find peace with each other. There is always some point to life, however pointless it may seem to the person living that life.

I mentioned that I had lunch with Gill and Peter Berryman on Saturday. In the early 1970s, they had a number of au pairs, one of whom was Elisabeth. After she'd left them, she used to return for a week or so each year, and in 1975, Peter, who was also the coach at Rosslyn Park, told me and Elisabeth independently that he had decided he had found the person we should respectively marry. Elisabeth, aged 24, and I, 28, had an arranged marriage. Peter and Gill introduced us at the Ponte Vecchio restaurant in the Old Brompton Road one Saturday evening. At the end of the week, Elisabeth went home to Seefeld, but, being a good boy and girl, we did what the coach told us. We married two years later, on 22 January 1977.

Gill has four children, of each and every one of whom

she is, as all mothers are, hugely proud. For the last year or two, Gill has had what was diagnosed initially as irritable bowel syndrome. It wasn't. It was bowel cancer. Slashed, but too late; it had spread to her liver. Chemotherapy shrunk the new tumour, slashed again two weeks ago. She will need some more chemo just to clear out any traces that the knife may have missed. Gill also had a pulmonary embolism and is on warfarin.

I call in some mornings to Peter and Gill's house in Kingston after being on the river, and we have a cup of tea and a natter about deep and meaningful stuff like the price of fish. If I've forgotten to take my warfarin that morning, she gives me some of hers. Which is very kind of her, as I don't want to boast but every day I take 15 mg, which is three times her daily dosage.

On Saturday lunchtime, Gill was looking good and eating huge portions; she's gonna be fine.

The other thing about this weekend was that I realised that, as I am now just carrying on with life, after six months, wherever I go, having cancer is no longer a problem for me or the people I'm with. People know about it, but as I seem to be physically pretty much the same, it's not even a point of conversation. Everyone has their own concerns, which quite often they talk about to me. I like it and listen. It seems lots of guys are having DREs or PSA tests. They tell me about it. I listen. As I found out quite early on, people will take their cue from me.

Sometimes, I am not so saintly. On Saturday, I go to support my team, Rosslyn Park. My blood is on the pitch, I know the exact spots where I broke my knee and did many other things, and I remain endlessly supportive and enthusiastic. So when we are having a bad patch at twenty-five minutes to four and I'm still chirping away, one of my old, well-established friends, who is a little taciturn and would be a good replacement for the grumpy guy in the Rising Sun in St Mawes, says, slightly critically, 'You'll still be shouting for the team when we're in the Surrey League, Division 5.'

'No I won't,' I say, 'because I'll be dead.' Very naughty.

Perhaps, as Sylvia Plath put it in 'New Year on Dartmoor', I want the world in a glass hat.

Thursday, 8 December 2005

I'm sitting in my room at 4.30 in the afternoon, and it is pitch black outside. Just two weeks to the winter solstice. I can see nothing in the window apart from my reflection. Gorgeous. I know Ho Chee's trees are out there beyond the reflection. It makes me feel happy. The big Wellingtonia, the copper beech, which has long since lost all its leaves, although, strangely, the beech tree is still wearing its crinkling russet autumn cloak.

Over the last three days, I've been eating for Britain. Today, I had a wonderful lunch, and spoke at the Merchant Taylors' Hall in Threadneedle Street to about 50 members of the City Forum. We were in one of those old wood-panelled guildhall rooms with their huge chandeliers. It was a privilege just to be in the room. I got invited because I used to play rugby, appeared on the TV for a few moments in *Superstars* and, for about 30 years, shuffled about around EC3 earning a crust. Actually, probably the real reason I was asked is that I don't charge and I happened to be in when the phone went. I mentioned earlier that Sandy Saunders, our England tour manager, very much old school, said to the team after the New Zealand tour in 1973, 'Boys, you'll dine out on this for the rest of your life.' As I said, I didn't know what he meant then, but I do now.

It was the first time I'd spoken at an event since I got

diagnosed. It has opened up a new line in material. This is another side benefit. For some reason which I really can't explain, people seem to be not so much interested but rather entertained by me just recounting the events of June 2005. Although I must admit I didn't find them that funny at the time. When I tell them that a PSA over 5 is a concern and over 10 a real worry but that mine was a gold-medal-winning you-are-toast 133, it seems to bring the house down. Yep, people will take their cue from you: treat it as a bit of a laugh and so will they. And so they should and so will I, for as long as I can.

Yesterday was Elisabeth's birthday. All the kidlets were away, but with my new feminine side, I knew what to do. Flowers – lilies and gypsophila – and a card bought and written with thought. Get up, make a special effort, white tablecloth, candles, carols and porridge. (Yep, porridge. She likes it! She is from the mountains, after all.) Coffee, toast, one slice for Torben. Then I had booked a lunch at Newick Park, Elisabeth's favourite place.

In the meantime, after breakfast, I drove up to the Marsden in Sutton, just over 20 miles in about 35 minutes, not too far, parked the car (I've now got the car-parking system sussed). Everyone here at the Marsden is brilliant, although I've obviously got particularly high expectations about my doctor, since he's the gatekeeper to a cure, and he hasn't indicated to me yet whether he's gonna unlock the door.

I get lost in the maze of buildings and go into the Cancer Research Centre to ask for directions at the reception desk. I can't help but notice a board with a notice about a meeting at 11.00 entitled 'Hot Issues in Prostate Cancer'.

Bizarre, really. I've often been in quasi-academic environments and the Cancer Research Centre was just such a place. I wonder if those guys going to the meeting know how keen we in the Club are that they should really, I mean really, pay attention. Or are they like I've always been in such situations: probably turn up late, give half an ear and drift out early if it's dull. Pay attention, you white coats, and sort it out for us on the wire.

Eventually, I find the blood-test room. I take my number from the machine and wait my turn. I notice two things: how old we all are, in our comfortable chairs, and how brave we all are, pretending to be so much better than we probably really are – polite, friendly, scared but, above all, brave. We're making light of the situation, like when you fall over and pretend it never really happened and smile on the outside while doing a double wince on the inside. We brave little soldiers never cry.

Well, having the blood sample taken is of course no big medical deal. It is the thought that on 14 December those few drops of blood will indicate how my PSA has changed since 7 September and will give me and the doctors the information to decide on the next step. Forwards? Or backwards?

However, the crucial thing is the same as it has been ever since I was diagnosed: don't think about it, put it to one side, live your life and enjoy your life. Don't waste your time worrying, eat a hearty breakfast, blah, blah, blah. You know the script by now.

Elisabeth and I have a wonderful lunch, it's her day, we drive home.

As I say, I am eating for Britain, as on 6 December, we had a Christmas lunch for DHSM, a syndicate management company for whom I'm a non-exec director. Earlier that morning, en route for the lunch, I'd made a play for the teaching job at PWC. It would be nice to get it, but as with all these things, you just have to give it your best shot. Everyone's got their own agendas. We'll see. If I get it, great; if I don't, move on. Anyway, there could be a conflict if I'm put on the list for radiotherapy, as that's six weeks out. Still, there are bridges other than Anxiety Bridge and I needn't cross them yet either.

Tomorrow is Mum's birthday. Ever since she died the whole family has got together on the weekend nearest her birthday, and tomorrow is the first day of this year's family do.

Friday, 9 December 2005

I nip up to Mum's grave and light a candle. She was born 96 years ago today. No one loves you like your mum loves you.

I come home, take Torben for a walk and do an easy 6,000 m on the ergometer. I've decided not to really hurt myself. I average 1 min. 59 sec. per 500 m and finish in just under 24 minutes. Better to just do something than to go all out, hurt myself and literally put myself off for life.

Mum was born in 1909 in Lincoln and in a different world, the eldest daughter of Joseph Pickering (1875–1956) and Jessie, née Holloway (1877–1938). They lived in a house called Wynberg in Cherry Willingham, then a village, now a suburb of Lincoln. Mum's sister Leah (1912–1971) was born three years later.

Joseph Pickering worked as a tradesman in Ruston & Hornsby engineering works in Lincoln, but the big influence in his life was a stint in the army in South Africa in 1901–2. He seems to have been a sensitive man and was horrified at what he saw, particularly the treatment of the Boer prisoners. Jackie, my sister, said that he became a conscientious objector as a result.

Mum always spoke fondly of Cherry and how life had been almost idyllic, describing cycling the three miles to

South Park Girls School, skating on the Witham when it froze over in winter and the wisteria around the house. She enjoyed all forms of sport, particularly tennis and hockey. Mum was always proud of the fact that she played hockey for Lincolnshire County Girls. Wherever we lived, she always belonged to a tennis club and, through the church, the Women's Institute. Both Mum and her sister were scholarship girls and loved school and learning, which is why they both went to teacher training college, probably one of the few opportunities not then denied to bright young working-class women.

Mum did her training in Tottenham, and her first teaching post was in Sheffield. She met Dad, I imagine, in the early 1930s, but I know it was on a train from Sheffield to Lincoln. Dad was travelling from Liverpool, where he was a marine engineer working for the White Star Line. I think he was quite good looking and spent his money on smart clothes and cars. In the downturn of the 1930s, he must have been quite a catch. They married on 2 November 1937. Leah said it broke their mother's heart, but Mum said our grandmother had been butted by a cow when she was crossing a field, that this brought on stomach cancer, and that this was what killed her in 1938, not a broken heart. Anyway, it was obviously not a match made in heaven.

With Dad on leave every two years from dodging Hitler's nautical hordes, by 1947 there was Mickey, Jackie, Lois, Eileen and finally me. By the time I was seven, Mum had decided that things were not as they should be in her life. I don't think there were any particular incidents or violence or even unpleasantness, but maybe there were. I don't really know why my mum decided to leave my father (they never divorced; maybe it was a late-1940s generational thing), but she must have had her reasons. My dad, I do know, was referred to as 'the ogre'. What effect did it have on us children? Well, Mickey moved to London not long after they separated; Jackie was always strong, and circumstances later in her life were to make her stronger. Apparently, Dad was unkind to Lois, Eileen has been a bit scarred by what happened, and I was too young to remember anything other than the food parcels, chocolate and cod-liver oil (shudder) he always brought for us. I think my mum left my dad for us children, to give us a better life, which she thought, rightly or wrongly, we would have without him. Mum, I know, would never put herself before any one of her children individually let alone collectively. She legally separated from my dad in 1955.

We then lived at 86 Elm Hall Drive, Allerton, Liverpool, and I can remember cycling on my trike to the Martin's Bank at the end of the road and going down the back entry to stand on the iron bridge at Mossley Hill above the smoke of the steam trains on the four tracks that passed below. We lived there until 1956 and then a few things happened. Mickey, at 16, left school – Quarry Bank, the same place John Lennon went to. Mickey says he does remember him. Crumbs, Mick, there's a John Lennon industry out there. Just another Liverpool scally, with Yoko claiming the rights over his death and, by the look of things in my local bookshop, Cynthia over his birth. Who cares? The rest of us have got his music. Mick went to work in London, in the road-accident statistics section of the civil service. Leah's husband died young. So Mum, Leah and their dad decided to buy a house in Bristol. Mick could come home and go back to school.

Mum's dad, Joseph, lived with us at 8 Belvedere Road, Redland, Bristol, for just a short while. He was 82 and had colon cancer. He had, from his perspective, seen his two daughters and his grandchildren together, safe and with a roof over our heads. He was in pain, and his time had come. He must have planned it with the skill of an engineer. He gassed himself on Thursday, 18 December 1956 in the cellar of Belvedere Road. I think, before the use of non-toxic North Sea gas, toxic coal gas was often chosen as a way to commit suicide. Jackie found his body, covered him, turned off the gas tap and opened the windows. She was 15.

I know it was a Thursday because that was the day *The Eagle* comic came out, four and a half old pence. Being the youngest, I never got to see it first, but that day I did. I remember feeling very detached, nine and almost otherworldly. Is that how we deal with death?

Mum loved us all and devoted her life to us. She carried on teaching, but money was, I imagine, an issue, although not as big a one as it could have been, as my dad always sent money and regularly long, long letters from faraway ports. Apart from one brief occasion, I didn't see him again till I was 22.

Mum always encouraged us in everything. We children owe a huge debt to Mum, which, now she is no longer with us, we are repaying in part by carrying on her values, her kindness, and living them for her grandchildren to see.

Elisabeth and I arrive at Longleat Center Parcs at 3.00 p.m. The weekend starts here. Rock on.

Saturday, 10 December to Monday, 12 December 2005

Center Parcs: two words, two deliberate spelling mistakes and a concept.

The concept is to create heaven on earth for any ten-year-old boy. Flumes, plumes, mountain bikes and everything with chips. If you're a ten-year-old boy with, say, an elder brother of twelve, a sister about eight, a dad who plays hockey and a mum who did triathlons and will do again when she eventually has some time to herself, and some of your ten-year-old friends have got their families to come along as well, if that's you, get on down to your nearest Center Parcs, 'cause it was built for you and it'll be the best few days of your life.

There were 45 of us bonding: 5 siblings (58–66) and partners, 15 children (19–42) and some partners and 10 grandchildren, squeaking (0–3 plus Jesse, 18) spread over 8 villas (well, more like Portakabins actually, but well fitted out).

Don, who is kindly and married to my sister Jackie and was/is an Oxford don and is 80 did not have the greatest three days of his life. Except, one lunchtime in Huckleberry's, in the 28°C dome, eating the sort of food you would imagine you'd eat in a place called Huckleberry's, Don suddenly heard a real jazz band playing the stuff he had loved when he too had played in a jazz band. He now thinks that, even for him (quite frankly a completely flume-free zone), Center Parcs is not complete rubbish.

I won't go into it all, other than to say that this year the family is growing exponentially: three births. Eleanor to Joe and Emma; Isaac, a son adopted by Anna and Paul; and Eva, a daughter for Vicki, who had just got married to her Cuban lover Jovi. Lucy brought her boyfriend Neil, who is a Welsh ex-shepherd, now doing a PGCE. Well, you get the drift, everyone seemed to have a great time, and there is an ugly rumour we may be back next year. Maybe not me!

Anyway, the prospect of 14 December faded into the background.

Tuesday, 13 December 2005

Back in my own bed, in cosy land. What a relief. No time to dawdle, today is a busy day. Up at 7.30 to cook the porridge that Marcus doesn't want. He is turning into a big unit, about 6 ft 5 in. and 17 st., and he found out in Dubai he can run quick. He is monosyllabic in the mornings and has an aversion to adverbs. Elisabeth loves him to bits. She definitely isn't monosyllabic and likes giving him advice, which, obviously, he doesn't actually want, and buying him shoes he'll never wear. He's a polite boy and loves his mum and pretends to listen to her good advice on what could be, as far as he is concerned, the price of eggs in Karlsruhe. The good advice is usually about not going outside with wet hair or wearing a coat – sensible, good, kind mum stuff. He probably would actually listen if it was advice about the price of eggs in Karlsruhe. They go to the station. I take Torbs for a three-mile wander. It's unusually warm. It hasn't rained for ages, but the tracks are still muddy. No other dog walkers are about. Torben will soon be in the old Hunderheim for Christmas. Poor old Torbs. Back home, Stef is up and on her way back to Norwich. I have a second breakfast, then wave goodbye and head off to Lingfield Surgery for an INR blood check (all fine at 2.2) and another 28-day injection of Zoladex, my seventh.

Get home, do a 19-minute pyramid erg, have a bath and then get on the good old 11.44 heading up to Victoria and Green Park Tube and Langan's for lunch at 12.45.

For the last five years or so, five of us – Christopher Wayne Ralston, Roger Uttley, Tony Neary, Jan Webster and me – have met for Christmas lunch. Thirty-two years ago, we were a third of the team that beat the All Blacks in New Zealand. As their lives have moved on, the others seem uninterested when I bore them with the fact that we were the only home country to have defeated New Zealand at home in the entire twentieth century. Wayne looks at me from behind his fading eyes, two hip replacements and two wives down the line from that victory, and says something along the lines of, 'We played five other games on that tour, we lost four and "smashed" Fiji 13–12, so maybe we weren't so brilliant.'

They seem more interested in my libido or lack of it and how this seems to make me more attractive to women, rather like a eunuch in a harem. Quarter to one turns into quarter to seven. We'll do it again next year. Nero says, 'Do we book for four or five?' Why do I find this so hilarious?

We have also agreed, as far as I can remember, to cycle across America, all go and live in Spain, visit a fair in Northumberland, go skiing (for some reason, on 22 March) and go to the Turks and Caicos Islands. Good old Langan's house red.

Wednesday, 14 December 2005

Up early, as I want to write about how I feel before my appointment at the Marsden at two, because afterwards I may have a completely different perspective. But, now, I'm feeling good – strong physically and mentally. Good news or bad, I'll cope. At least, I think I will. Who knows? Not much to add to what I've already said. I feel sort of detached, like when I was reading *The Eagle* just after my grandfather committed suicide. Is this how I handle death? Is this how I will handle my death? When in due course it comes. But not yet, Lord, please not yet. My shoulder aches.

I've just checked through my emails, and I've received one from Rob Cornford telling me that Richard Sandbrook,

59, who had been at the UEA reunion on Saturday, 17 September, died of cancer on 11 December. Our reunion was just ten weeks ago. We chatted with each other, and he never mentioned he had cancer. He must have known, he must have known then it was terminal. He seemed to be having a great time. He'd been president of the Students' Union, loved intrigue and gossip, smoked, drank, schemed, he was always thin, Mary loved him, always looked as if he needed a scrub and polish, very bright, I never met his children. I reckon he had a good time till 11 December.

UEA's motto was 'Do different', and Richard had indeed done different. He had a social conscience, was a big wheel first in Friends of the Earth then in other Good Works stuff. In the Club, there are no rules as to how you handle it. We each have our own way, and each way is perfect. Rest in peace Richard. You had a good and fulfilled life, and what more can any of us hope for?

I'll write no more till maybe this evening, but I'll think about a friend and the grief of his family. I'll pray for them and all of us.

Later, Wednesday, 14 December 2005

My PSA has fallen over the last three months from 1.1 to 0.8. I don't know why but I almost feel guilty. Today, I haven't anything else to add or say.

Thursday, 15 December 2005

So far, so very lucky, but no false hopes, no Anxiety Bridge. Feet on the ground, whatever comes at you, just deal with it. Then put it to one side and get on with the wonderful business of living.

However this is how it has been for me so far.

PART TWO

A suspected heart attack in the morning of 5 June 2005. It wasn't, it was a couple of blood clots in my lungs – a pulmonary embolism. Great and quick treatment from East Surrey Hospital, Saint Shrilla and Dr Sneddon gave me all the tests to find out what caused it. Probably it was a cocktail of locally advanced cancer in the prostate, a recent severe attack of phlebitis and maybe a genetic leaning (my sister Eileen had a PE when she was pregnant). Who knows? However, six months of warfarin has prevented any further embolisms and helped clear up my varicose veins. Maybe I'll go and see Dr Sneddon soon and perhaps come off the warfarin.

The really lucky bit came during the investigation in East Surrey Hospital. Saint Shrilla asked for a PSA test to be made, which is not always done for a PE. It was my good fortune, because if she hadn't done the test then, now, on Friday, 15 December 2005, I would not have a dog's chance of a cure, which I believe I have.

The PSA test is a far from perfect test, particularly as some prostate-cancer tumours will not generate a huge amount of PSA. So it is possible (estimated as high as a 20 per cent chance) to have a low (say, under 4 ng/ml) PSA score and yet still have an aggressive cancer (even a Gleason 8 or above). However, the higher the PSA, the less likely the error. An initial PSA above 20 probably indicates a cancer that is outside the window of opportunity for surgery. Most cancers which cause a PSA result above 70 are still treatable but not curable. My initial PSA score was 133 ng/ml.

The question was not whether it had spread outside the prostate gland but how far it had spread. A bone scan showed the cancer was not in my bones. An MRI scan indicated it might have spread to my lymph nodes, but not necessarily. It just might have. I had great treatment

243

at East Surrey Hospital. Even though according to the NHS reporting tables at the time, they ticked few of the boxes, for me, they ticked every box.

Radiotherapy was not offered to me, but unlike surgery it was a distant possibility. With both surgery and radiotherapy, unless they address the complete problem and there is a good chance of a cure, don't bother. If the cancer has spread beyond the scope of surgery and/or radiotherapy then there is little point in having a spreading disease accompanied, for no real benefit, by the side effects of surgery and/or radiotherapy.

This was exactly my unequivocal position on 25 June 2005.

Like most locally advanced and advanced prostate-cancer sufferers, I was put on low-dose Casodex (50 mg) for 30 days to prevent flare, and after about 10 days, I had my first injection of Zoladex.

To date, I have been fortunate in that I have reacted well to this treatment, which defers but does not cure prostate cancer. It extends the piece of string, and there can be a range of side effects. For most patients, the big concern is loss of libido; for me, it is the reduction in my performance on the ergometer. Sad. We are all winged in some way. It can be many years before the cancer cells become Zoladex resistant (usually marked by a sustained PSA bounce). Even then, other stuff can be done.

My good fortune is that my cancer has to date responded well to the hormone treatment, and this has resulted in a reduced PSA count. First test, 15 June: 133. Second, 14 July: 95. Third, 17 August: 3.2. Fourth, 12 September: 1.1. Fifth, 14 December: 0.82.

The doctor has decided to let the process of degrading the cancer cells through the use of Zoladex continue and has made an appointment in a further three months' time, on 15 March 2006. I believe that if the PSA has stayed low, the hospital will give me IMRT radiotherapy over a wide pelvic area, as they believe that, with a 133 initial PSA score, there will be degraded but not dead cancer cells that are hormone resistant but not IMRT resistant still well spread around the pelvic area.

The IMRT is part of a test being run by the Marsden. They have also asked me to stay on hormone treatment for three years. Still, this is making assumptions that I am in no position to make. I'm feeling good, although my shoulder still sort of hurts. I am lucky. Each day is a gift, and for no reason I can think of, today, right now, I am feeling like a hero.

Saturday, 17 December 2005

For the last day or so, for the best and maybe even the worst of reasons, I've been thinking about Richard Sandbrook. We never even knew each other that well, but our paths crossed kindly, albeit not much and not that often, at UEA and in the 35 years after. We never sought each other out, but I always had the feeling he liked me as I liked him. I gave him a lift once from Norwich to somewhere in Gloucestershire, and he, in spite of his dirty fingernails and comfortable background, had bucketloads of sensible empathy for the world. He fell in love with Mary. Then again, most of us fell in love with Mary, if only from afar. Strangely, it seemed to me, she fell in love with him, and always and only with him. She must now be hurting, empty, missing him, her constant friend, companion and love.

I feel for him and his family, but it's not just that, which is good and kind. Yes, it's not just that. It's far worse than just that.

I have become so self-obsessed, so self-concerned – not actually selfish but just utterly preoccupied with me. So I think about Richard and how his death relates to me. Well, of course, it doesn't. I can't even begin to know or understand how his whole family must feel. Numb, strong – such a mass of emotions that I can't imagine.

I had assumed, apparently wrongly, that when I saw him last, on 17 September, he must have known about his cancer. It seems he didn't.

Imogen was at UEA at the same time, beautiful, like Mary, although she had fallen for Laurie Heritage. Laurie was like James Dean, except blonder, brooding, though, and he too had what seemed to me like more than just superficial personal hygiene issues. He, unlike Richard, was crazy, not just obsessively reading Isaac Asimov, keeping motorbike bits in a box in his room type of crazy (although he was that) but genuinely crazy. Anyway, Imogen had been at the same reunion on 17 September. She has married a vampire – well, someone from Transylvania – and lives outside Vienna. She told me about Richard.

Richard didn't know about his cancer on 17 September, which is why he didn't speak about it. He did know that he had had a heart attack earlier in the year and was taking drugs for that. When all his limbs started aching, he thought it was the drugs that were doing it. He also knew that he had had a melanoma removed three years ago. During October 2005, despite a change of drugs, the aches and pains didn't get any better, so, taking another tack, the white coats discovered cancer in his bones and, much more seriously, a couple of lesions on his brain and spine. Presumably, these were secondary cancers from the original melanoma. Five weeks, just five weeks.

So what can I do? Well, first of all, I can try to get better, and I can try to use the bit of extra string, however long that is, to make a difference. How can I do that? Well, I can get this story published and give the proceeds, if there are any, to cancer research. I can write not just for me but for others like me, who are also some way down the prostate-cancer curve. We are not alone, as, importantly, those at the beginning, who have just been told they have prostate cancer, may be able to find hope in those of us who have already made or are making the journey they are about to embark on. Having been a guest of the NHS for the last six months or so, I now know that if you are gonna get cancer, there has never been a better time than now, and the earlier it's detected the more can be done. Bye, Richard. I'll run hard for you and me and the rest of the Club.

Saturday morning, weak sun, cold, no wind, getting light at 7.45, up to Richmond Lock from Chiswick in a coxless four. My loss of strength is not so obvious in a boat as it is on the ergometer. In fact, I think I'm rowing better. Maybe I'm pulling clever, not ripping up the water and not, even at my current weight, destabilising the boat. Maybe I'm feeling the water better, like female rowers often do. So that's yet another benefit of Zoladex.

Back to the clubhouse. Nigel, the *Daily Mail* photographer is there with his camera. For the last three Saturdays, when I've been at Tideway Scullers, there has also been a photographer. My fellow oarsmen think this is somehow amusing. I tell them it's because I'm a famous star and they're not. This goes down very well. Actually, I love the attention. So that's yet another benefit of Zoladex.

Cup of tea, up to Rosslyn Park for an ex-players' Christmas reunion lunch as Crampo's guest. Crampo, where does one start? Well, better if we don't go down that route. Forty years has taught me that if you follow

Cramp you'll finish up eating pickled eggs, hitting yourself over the head with a plate with no clothes on, trying to avoid flying furniture and throwing up. Rosslyn Park smash North Walsham 27–25, I slip away. Learning to slip away, that's yet another benefit of Zoladex.

That's three nil.

Oh, yes, I almost forgot: today, I also learned about perspective, about how we all see things from a different angle, even if we are looking at the same thing; there are probably as many perspectives on that same thing as there are pairs of eyes. At the Rosslyn Park Christmas lunch, sitting next to Crampo on his left-hand side is his brother-in-law Brett. I'm on Crampo's right-hand side and Gonzo is opposite him. There are ten or so of us at this long trestle table. There are about ten tables crammed into the bar and the chef and staff are doing Christmas miracles with the lunch and sprigs of holly.

Gonzo is now 53. He was diagnosed with prostate cancer at a private company health check when he was 48, with a PSA rising from 4 to 7 over two years, a positive DRE and a Gleason score 6. Almost immediately following the biopsy, he had a radical prostatectomy. Gonzo woke up from the general anaesthetic without a prostate gland but with both a catheter and an erection. He is the least winged of anyone I know who has had a radical prostatectomy. He had short-term incontinence and blood in the urine but the bonus of a negligible PSA. The only medium/long-term consequence of having no prostate is that Gonzo can have an orgasm but he has no ejaculate. This is apparently not a problem, and he and his wife save on cleaning bills. There is also, I understand, another potential side effect of surgery, which is that as the urethra goes through the prostate, it may be pulled up. As the urethra then goes through the penis, this pulling up can diminish its size. Gonzo assures me this is not true, at least not in his case. Last summer, he did the Étape du Tour stage of the Tour de France. He still has six-monthly checks but has, to all intents and purposes, moved on. Get it early and Gonzo's is the result you can hope for. He is very sympathetic to me.

Brett, aged 45, had a pulmonary embolism about the same time, in June 2005, as I did. He went into hospital, was put on heparin then on warfarin, with regular weekly then fortnightly checks. He has taken the tablets (12 mg) at the same time each day, but his INR has ranged from 1.6 to 3.9. Consequently, he has sensibly been careful about diet and alcohol intake. He was not drinking at the Christmas lunch, and, surprisingly, Crampo left him alone. Perhaps it wasn't too surprising, really. Brett is Jo's (Mrs Crampo's) brother, and in this world only she can instil fear into the Cramp.

Me, I've almost forgotten about my PE. I make sure I remember to take the warfarin. Although PE kills 30,000 in the UK each year and prostate cancer 10,000, with PE it's usually quick: blood clot, breathless, gone. With most cancers, if you don't get rid of them, then it's a piece of string along the length of which life is drawn out of you. So unlike Brett, because that may be my future, I'm determined to enjoy life, and as a consequence, I have made few concessions as regards either diet or drink. I know this is stupid, but 'Eat, drink and be merry, for tomorrow we die' has lots of resonance for me at the moment.

In a way, this difference of perspective is like one's attitude to getting up to go to the lavatory at night. Some of us get up, say, twice a night and consider this to be a pretty good deal, while others would regard it as an intolerable imposition. I suppose the ultimate cliché about perspective is 'Is the glass half empty or half full?' Me, I'm firmly in the half-full camp.

Before I move on, this whole peeing business is now a fact of life for me. As yet, I haven't experienced incontinence; I'm just in the foothills, whereas for those suffering from BPH, peeing is the major factor affecting the quality of their life. How do you deal with this? I don't know and have little advice. All I can say is how it is for me, a 58-year-old man with locally advanced prostate cancer.

I seem to have bladder control. Occasionally, perhaps once a month, I may get an urgent need to pee. It is usually not a traumatic experience. Most of the time during the day, I notice no difference from when I was a younger man. At night, it depends, I imagine, on how long I sleep and how much liquid I drink. There are also other variables, but generally there is a gap between about two and six hours, so on average this is a pee about every four hours. So if I am in bed for less than seven hours, I'll get up on average once. Some nights can be better or worse than others, and I am not too sure why. When I broke my ribs, the walk to the lavatory – same floor, about 40 ft away – was unbelievably painful. I didn't walk. I put a screwtop bottle by the bed. For some reason, I didn't like this. However, at present, in my current list of concerns, if dying is one and the price of fish is ten, then urination worries are about eight. Lucky me.

There are two other things I'll mention in passing about peeing. First, because I don't put the light on at night when I go to the lavatory, I don't have a strong stream and I am not circumcised, sometimes I pee down my leg or on my pyjama trousers. So now I sit down to pee. Unless my knees hurt and it is a low bowl. Second, when I sit down to pee, because I'm putting fat on my pubic bone, my penis seems to have shrunk, and unless I point it down, I pee between the toilet seat and the bowl.

Thought I'd mention this because, well, we now know

each other well enough to talk about these things, and who else is going to tell you about this stuff, which, if you're in the Club, prostate branch, you may know about already.

The way to make a friend, apparently, is to say three kind things about someone and then tell them a confidence. Well, you've just had a confidence from me, so I reckon you and I are now friends. Oh, yes, just in case no one has ever told you, you are kind, you are brave, and you, especially you, deserve better. Now we really are friends. 'Cause that's how it works.

Sunday, 18 December 2005

Last rowing outing of this year: sunny, cold and it's getting light at about 7.55. We are going out in an eight. We wait for the light. River ebbing, halfway towards low tide. This is the first time I've been out in an eight since early spring, another place, another life away. After single sculls and pairs and fours, an eight seems like a battleship. In fact, my weight is more than the entire 60-ft shell and all the trimmings. I sit stroke side, number four, in the middle. It's an experienced crew, the battleship is a forgiving companion, we row well. I haven't the words to tell you how good it feels to be in an eight, gliding across the flat water, with almost minimum effort, flowing, racing, relaxing, stronging, stealthing along in harmony. We are all invincible, we will all live forever, poems will be written about us and our great-grandchildren will be told of our outing this crispy, glorious, forever-golden Sunday morning.

Get home. Stef and Mouse and Bryony (they now seem to be joined at the hip) are ready for lunch. Gill (slashed two weeks ago and awaiting further chemo) and Peter Berryman join us with their daughter Tamsyn. Sunday lunch: what a brilliant meal. Elisabeth gives it an Austrian flavour. I am drinking too much. I must be doing a bottle of wine a day. I like it. And to think up until I was 40 I never really drank alcohol. We are all happy. Not surprising, if we are doing a bottle of wine each. The afternoon gurgles on. Log fire, late-afternoon walk, this is idyllic.

That evening, Elisabeth and I go to the Christmas carol concert at St John's. Amen.

Tuesday, 20 December 2005

The Range Rover, now with 152,000 miles on the clock and following a wash and brush-up from Mr Tovey, takes us to Dover to be in time for the 7.00 a.m. Sealink ferry. On the ferry, eating a cross-channel heart-stopper of a breakfast and looking out of the restaurant window, I can just make out the dark foreboding rollers. Some 25 degrees south of the Sealink ferry, on about latitude 25 degrees north and about 23 degrees west, 30 or so seagoing rowing boats are crossing the Atlantic, three weeks out of the Canary Isles. For the crews, it will be like spending between 40 and 100 days in a washing machine. Now, with four days of picking up the afterwash of Hurricane Epsilon, they will have the bonus effect of a spin dryer added in. There are two singles in the race. In one is a woman, Roz Savage. Why? We human beings are strange.

With Sealink, it's a one-way fare of £50 for all of us and our Christmas presents. Mouse is working, but will join us on 24 December. Eurotunnel is advertising a £49 one-way deal but seems, for the time we want to train it, to be in triple-digit land, as does P&O. Norfolkline might be worth a look, but the Range doesn't know the way from Boulogne. It knows: Calais, Brussels, Liège, Aachen, Köln, Koblenz, Ludwigshafen, Karlsruhe, Stuttgart (great airport), München, Scharnitz and, finally, Seefeld. 700 miles: 10 hours at 70 mph with 2 stops. We get there at 9.00 p.m. Elisabeth is home again.

There is an article about me in the *Daily Mail* today, by Marianne Power; it is kind. This is the third article in about as many weeks, following Paul Kimmage's in the *Sunday Times* and Mick Cleary's in the *Daily Telegraph*. Since Paul's article, I've moved from the sport pages to the health pages. Actually, the name strikes me as inaccurate, as the health sections of most newspapers are all about not-health and people's brave fights against crippling, malignant diseases. My story, for the moment, seems to fit the bill. Like the obituary column, the not-health section seems to be a growth area in most newspapers.

In my pomp, 30 years ago, I used to get self-conscious about being in the newspapers, probably something to do with the embarrassment of recognising the fact that I am an attention-seeking self-publicist. Now I know it'll all pass pretty quickly, but maybe as a result one more man will go and get a DRE, and that makes me feel good.

Wednesday, 21 December 2005

The winter solstice. The sun is at right angles to the tropic of Capricorn at 23.5 degrees south; the earth is now rotating back towards the tropic of Cancer, but it's OK, 'cause it means the sun is also coming back to the northern hemisphere and even to me here in Seefeld.

When, after 25 June 2005, I was desperately organising my life in view of my then imminent death, Elisabeth and I decided we would have to sell Ho Chee's house, so she could buy a small flat in London for the kidlets, we'd do up the two-bedroomed flat here in Seefeld, and Elisabeth could live off the cash left over. It would work. I didn't die, and we didn't sell Ho Chee's house, but we did do up the flat. We have just arrived; Herr Gapp, the carpenter, has refurbished it as a *Stube*, with full wood panelling. It is a two-bedroomed palace. It is magnificent. We are now, as Clouds says, living in a tree. Elisabeth is so happy to be home.

Thursday, 22 December 2005

She has come back to have a little chat – more than I did for Moya. But she's obviously more considerate than I was, and, it seems, she's got a deal for me.

Each morning in the mountains is magic. Surrounded by the towering Seefelderspitze and Seefelderjoch, with the Hohe Munde behind, Seefeld sits on a 3,000-ft-high plateau. The snow is piled up high, and the yellow snowploughs with their huge friendly tyres, probably driven by our friend Bianca's dad and her brother Renee, clear the roads. There are 2,000 inhabitants waiting for the 10,000 guests that will explode onto this winter wonderland on 25 December after they have celebrated the coming of the Christkind in their own houses on Christmas Eve.

Now, today, it's all empty. It's magic.

I've been running and walking for 30 years through the pine forests that fill up most of the plateau. With my knees shot to bits, I can't alpine ski, so it's langlaufing for me. But in fact I prefer just walking. I know the surrounding hills well.

I set off for a walk at three o'clock, by myself. Elisabeth is enjoying the business of getting Christmas ready for us all. Actually, though, it's not Christmas. That was Mum and Bristol and brothers and sisters and getting up so early in the morning on 25 December and a pillowcase full of just everything and Christmas lunch, although we called it dinner then. Turkey and roast potatoes and all sorts of vegetables and stuffing and forcemeat balls, and afterwards Christmas pudding, with the hidden silver sixpence and a special only-at-Christmas custard. Then later a walk to Stoke Bishop to have Christmas dinner with Auntie Leah's best friend, Noel, who'd drive us home, and one year, when we were walking down Parry's Lane, it snowed. No, we are going to celebrate Weihnachten.

I step out towards Mosern, about 3 km away along the track by the Langlauf Weg, the cross-country skiing route. I am completely alone. In three days' time fur-coated Germany, and increasingly Russia, will have annexed this path. I head up the back route to the Moserer See and then cut across towards Wildmoss See. It's starting to get dark, but I know the path I am taking. The branches of the pine trees are so heavily laden with snow it's as if they have their hands by their sides. I am completely alone. I stop walking. It's snowing hard; there is absolutely no sound except for the noise of the snow as it falls on my jacket.

Now, if I was to see myself with the 30-years-ago eyes of a young man aged 28, what would I see? A friendly big nutter in the woods, head down, talking to himself?

Andrew, my love, remember I have never done you harm, and yet three weeks ago you said you wanted to kill me. How do you think I felt about that? Why are you so aggressive towards me? Although you are a man, you are not stupid, and I shouldn't have to repeat myself, but I will.

They have not tried to untangle me; they treat me as they treat others, but I am different, Andrew, I mean you no harm. We can live together. My love, they wish to turn us into both their meaningful subjects and docile objects. We can live together without them as one.

You can untangle me, Andrew, I am yours, I belong to you.

You can change me if you wish, but let us live together. I am powerful, you don't even begin to realise the power that will be yours, my love, if you let me live with you. We can do good, be good together for others.

Let the white coats continue with your treatment and they will blow away my shadow side, which I have never acknowledged. I will change for you, but don't kill me.

If this is a deal, what do I have to do for you?

Andrew, you are better than that. There is no deal. I am yours. Just let the changed me live in you. You can't even begin to imagine what we can do together. I ask nothing of you.

I get back to the inside of the magnificent tree. It's five o'clock, it's dark, and it's still snowing. I don't tell Stef and Clouds their dad has fruitcake potential, but I will. And what now is the young man of 28 saying? Maybe, 'Hey, matey, your choice but do you think it's wise for an old man on drugs to go walking by himself at dusk in the woods when it's snowing?'

Well, I can tell this young man how it is for this 58-year-old man with locally advanced prostate cancer, still in limbo land but now with prospects – just how it is. It is magic.

I am living today, the only day of value, with my wonderful family in an almost-tree on a forested, snow-covered plateau in an almost uninhabited, waiting village. The surrounding mountains are reaching for the sky, and so am I. Friends from afar tell me they love me, as I love them. The world could not be kinder. Elisabeth is back amongst her own, and to us she could not be more loving or happier. Clouds is playing with all the doors that may be open to her this summer. Stef is playing with a five-euro Wella blond hair kit, and Mouse will be here tomorrow and so will the Christkind. I am alive and strong and can walk 10 km through the woods with no ill effects. In my head, I have her and the Prostate Kid and now me at 28, but it is *me* tap-tap-tapping away. This is my tapping time. My magic time. My head is fine. We'll all be fine.

Friday, 23 December 2005

It has continued to snow hard during the night, and it is piling higher and higher. Today, somewhere out in the Atlantic, about 500 miles due west of the Canary Isles, Roz Savage is in a little boat by herself, and today is her birthday. I bet when she was younger she used to get joint Christmas and birthday presents, which is of course rubbish. That's usually the problem with having a birthday so near Christmas. Row on, Roz. Now, although we've never met, forgive me for saying it, it being your birthday 'n' all, but, Roz, you actually are the fruitcake.

I've decided to leave my head for a while and get back to the mechanics of medicine. I've now read and marked and notated the eight books about prostate cancer I bought on Amazon a few months ago.

Picking up from where I left off the last time I wrote about the medical mechanics, on 16 November, I am trying to add to my knowledge and am now beginning to look into radiation theory and in particular IMRT, as that is the type of radiation treatment I may be offered on 15 March 2006.

However, first off, **cell cycle time** seems worth a few thoughts.

An individual cell reproduces by dividing into two daughter cells (this is called mitosis). The cell cycle time is the time that elapses between a cell's division and the division in turn of the cells formed. Each type of cell has its own cycle time. Cells lining the mouth, for example, have a relatively short, 48-hour cycle time. Normal prostate cells often have a very long cycle time, as do some, but probably not all, prostate-cancer cells.

I am now on such thin ice as far as my medical knowledge goes that what I am about to write might be not just wrong, wholly or in part, but naive at best and dangerous at worst. But two thoughts.

First, a substance called spermine has been shown to inhibit the growth of prostate cancer. Spermine is found primarily in the prostate itself. Does this substance slow the growth of cancerous prostate cells (irrespective of whether they have a short or long cell cycle time) while those cells are encapsulated in the prostate? Maybe. However, once the cancer has spread and eventually advanced out of the prostate, the inhibiting effect of spermine is removed and the cancer then spreads rapidly compared to its growth rate in the prostate.

Second, if the cancerous cells in the prostate have a short cycle time, then, I imagine, the growth of the tumour will be a function of that cell cycle. So it follows rationally, but perhaps falsely, that those cancerous prostate cells with a long cycle time will move at a slower pace than those with a short cycle time.

External beam radiation therapy was developed in the 1950s using cobalt-60 radiation, which seemed to be as effective as surgery but carried with it its own set of adverse side effects. In the 1960s, linear accelerators allowed for bigger doses of radiation with relatively few side effects.

Radiation treatment, then and now, diminishes a cell's ability to undergo mitosis by damaging the cell's deoxyribonucleic acid – its DNA. Some cells die (apoptosis); they do not split. In uncontrolled amounts, radiation can be deadly, as it will kill off all sorts of normal cells. As a consequence, the side effects of radiotherapy can be substantial.

However, it has been found that most cancerous cells are less efficient in repairing radiation injury than normal cells. Some malignant tumours can be destroyed by amounts of radiation that have a lesser effect on normal cells.

So external beam radiation therapy, three-dimensional conformal radiation therapy, proton beam therapy and all their subsets are about controlling the radiation dose in order to kill off the cancerous cells and allow the normal cells to recover. IMRT, intensity-modulated radiation therapy, is just the latest development in radiotherapy, in which, hopefully, the side effects are now minimised. IMRT radiation therapists will custom-design a pattern and dose of radiation beams, with the objective of maximising the killing of cancer cells while minimising damage to normal tissue over as big an area as is warranted by the possible spread of cancer cells.

As I understand it, your individual IMRT treatment is devised by simulating the process with special X-rays to determine the dose and focus of radiation. Then I/you turn up every day, Monday to Friday, at the same time for seven weeks to have ten minutes of pre-programmed radiation treatment.

With external radiation treatment there is no surgery, no general anaesthetic, no transfusion risk, an impotence risk of about 35 per cent – the same as with surgery – incontinence is possible but unlikely (a 5 per cent risk) and there is usually no pain. Possible disadvantages include irritation of the bladder and rectum, and fatigue.

There is also continued debate as to whether radiation kills off all the cancerous cells or just stuns them. But does it matter if they are alive as long as they are inactive?

Here is my two pennyworths. To repeat myself, I am talking about something I know little about. Just to live the nightmare doesn't mean you understand it. However, before I continue, on this I am quite clear: cancer may not exactly be living the dream, but it is only a nightmare if you choose to make it that way. Cancer may take your body and ultimately your life, but it can never, ever own your heart or soul. They are yours and you can give them to whosoever you wish. We must find the hero inside ourselves. Then it's easier for us and for those who love us.

To continue, perhaps those prostate-cancer cells with a short cycle time, with, probably, aggressive growth characteristics, have their entire DNA energy focused on growth, not survival. These cancerous cells would then be apoptosised by radiation. Those cancerous cells with long cycles, however, might survive radiation but be impaired and take time to repair themselves, like some damaged normal cells. Does this matter? Maybe. However, if they are alive but inactivated, live with it and move on. Again, I must add this is a hypothesis on my part, a mere theory, a point of view based on no research.

One reason that the range of chemotherapy drugs, injected or in tablet form, are not used in early treatment of prostate cancer is that chemo drugs appear to be particularly efficient at apoptosising fast-growing cancer cells. This means that normal fast-growing cells, such as those in the lining of the mouth, the hair follicles, the lining of the gastrointestinal tract and the bone marrow, can also be temporarily affected by chemotherapy. This results in the side effects usually but not always associated with chemotherapy treatment, including mouth sores, loss of appetite, fatigue, hair loss, bleeding from minor injuries, diarrhoea and risk of infection. So chemotherapy as a front line treatment for the usually slow-moving prostate-cancer cells is not at this stage the treatment of choice, not because of the side effects but because hormonal therapy does a better job. It may be that if certain of the cancer cells become resistant to the hormonal treatment, then chemotherapy becomes an option. There are many cases of dramatic response to chemotherapy and I imagine that is when a characteristic of the cancer is when the cell has a short cell life. As yet these are not questions for me, but they are a reality for some further down the curve.

Having meandered through cell cycle time, I will in due course find out more about IMRT, in the knowledge that if I stay on the hormone treatment after the radiation treatment, even the degraded long-cycle cancerous cells may finally apoptosise. Sounds good to me, and that's the programme that I've agreed with the bouncy prof to be part of.

Saturday, 24 December and Sunday, 25 December 2005: Weihnachten

The Tyrol is in the west of Austria, an innately conservative, Catholic, Alpine land that has close ties with Bavaria in Germany and the South Tyrol in Italy, an ingrained suspicion of Vienna and, of course, a complete dislike of Switzerland. Each valley has a strong local identity, accentuated by its own localised dialect.

Austria is a country of about 8 million inhabitants, with a glorious political, military and especially cultural history, having been ruled for centuries by the great Habsburg dynasty. Before the Year of Revolution in 1848, when Germany, like Italy, was just a collection of dukedoms, independent provinces and states awaiting unification under Bismarck and Victor Emmanuel respectively, the Austro-Hungarian Empire, under the guidance of Metternich and Kaiser Franz Joseph, held sway in Central Europe. In 1914, Franz Joseph's nephew Archduke Franz Ferdinand was shot in Sarajevo. This event was to precipitate the First World War and bring about the rapid decline and division of the Habsburg Empire, a process that was finally completed after the 1939–45 war.

Vienna, a city of huge architectural and cultural significance, lost both its economic hinterland and its role as a communications hub. However, in the post-war era, the Tyrol, with its majestic Alpine landscape, has benefited massively, both culturally and economically, from the growth in winter sports.

Austria is a democratic socialist country where the hotel owner will have been to school with the waiter, where both will be concerned about high taxation but happy with the hospitals, education, public transport and social welfare provided by the state. Here, there is no social hierarchy as in the UK – after all, there has been a revolution. However, there is a shared underlying fear and concern about cultural invasion, and the recent lowering of border restrictions, has, if anything, heightened the ingrained intolerance of foreigners, different religions and different races.

Elisabeth is the eldest of five, two brothers and three sisters, and she is the only one of her enormous extended family (both her mother and father had seven brothers and sisters) to have left her home village and married a foreigner. After 30 years, and having helped drive the cows to milking on the high Alpine pastures in the summer, I am acknowledged as a member of the family.

Christmas here is traditional, of religious significance and fun. My children have only ever known this type of

Christmas, and in a minute I'll tell you all about what normally happens, although for us this year, Christmas 2005, it was slightly different.

OK. So far, so Kinder, Küche, Kirche. There is, however, just one other thing I should mention before unfurling these two days, and this is in no way judgemental, in fact, in my current state of non-libido, it is an observation made over almost 30 years and now grounded in envy. There is in Seefeld a lot of sex taking place, which ultimately, however tangentially, has an impact on most relationships. I believe this phenomenon is a post-war generational thing, and maybe a Seefeld-specific thing. I can almost count on one hand the number of relationships that have lasted the course here.

This is a holiday village with around 2,000 permanent inhabitants, plus another, say, 500 – usually Austrians from outside the high plateau, Serbians or Eastern Europeans – who work the winter season, which is from now for about 10 weeks. There are around 10,000 guests staying a week, which is about 100,000 visitors passing through each winter season. As the Americans say (and I find this expression mildly irritating, although nothing to get hung about, strawberry fields forever), 'Do the math.' Don't they know the shortened form of 'mathematics' is 'maths' not 'math'? Then again, would Americans get mildly irritated if we British were to say, 'Do the maths'?

Anyway, what do these 100,000 seasonal guests, who tend to be wealthy, want? These guests want sunshine, snow, skiing, snowboarding, saunas, swimming in hot pools, night skiing, fun, tradition, exclusivity, good food, pampering, casinos, nightclubs, sleigh rides, Alpine culture, shops, drink, yodelling, walking, to relax and to leave their day-to-day world with all its cares behind, to fall in love and have sex. Actually, that sounds like a good week to me. So the permanent inhabitants are like children in a sweet shop. I still can't work out why Elisabeth left.

Anyway, back to Weihnachten. Usually, at five in the evening on 24 December, we all sit down for a cold platter with a variety of meats and bread and gherkins and onions on a special white-linen cloth at the beautifully laid table. Christmas carols on the CD player and a good bottle of wine. We all love it. Then the father goes into the other room to check the angels have lit all the candles and turned out all the lights and that the Christkind has left presents under the Christmas tree. After this, the angels ring a bell, which is a sign to the children, who are washing their hands in the bathroom, that they should come into the other room. We all love it. Then the children read the story of the birth of Jesus; even Mouse (who, after a good Catholic education at Worth Abbey, is a confirmed atheist) takes his part. We then sing a couple of carols, even though none of us can sing. We unwrap the presents.

This is how it has been for the last 20 or more years, but this year was different.

Mouse, who had to work up until the 23rd, was catching an easyJet flight out of Stansted very early the following morning. He says he operates on a higher plane than most humans and so can be absent-minded. He forgot his passport. After lots of faffing about, at five o'clock in the evening on 24 December, Stef and I are not listening to Christmas carols on the CD player but driving to pick him up at Munich airport, which, as anyone who has used this airport knows, is just west of the Czech Republic. We took a five-hour time-out on Christmas this year, and so it started at ten o'clock instead. We still loved it.

Elisabeth does Christmas stockings on Christmas morning. At five in the evening, we go to the village church, the one Elisabeth and I got married in and where Mouse and

Clouds were baptised. Stef was baptised in Dormansland Church and is, like me, an Anglican Protestant. We then have the best meal of the year: a full turkey Christmas dinner, with Christmas pudding and everything.

We are blessed. I found myself a bit tearful, in the dark before the presents were opened, as we looked at the shimmering candles, lit by the angels, on the tree. Crying not like in Kalamata, and not for myself, just another sentimental old man grateful for so much, when so little is denied to so many. I feel a New Year's resolution coming on.

Thursday, 29 December 2005

I don't think I'm experiencing another knock-on effect of the hormone treatment, although emotional volatility is a characteristic side effect of Zoladex, it says so on the box. No, I think it's just something we all go through. There I was a few days ago, preparing to save the world, which I will still try to do – well, at least my teeny-weeny corner, my garden, my window box. Whereas today, I'm just pulling out of a slough of despond, brought on two days ago. So what happened two days ago?

Well, like most of humanity following a few days of excess, or, in my case, a few months of metaphorical mince pies, I was worried about putting on weight and not having enough money, probably in that order. Vanity before cash. The catalyst for this self-indulgent hitting the slough/trough phase was that Elisabeth, when out shopping with Stef and Clouds, put a small dent in another car while parking the Range Rover in the snowboard-shop car park in Innsbruck. She chose some guy called Torsten's top-of-the-range brand-new Mercedes.

Anyway, before we get into the money thing, the weight

thing. Because prior to denting Torsten's pride and joy, Elisabeth bought a pair of scales, because she knew I'd enjoyed weighing myself in East Surrey Hospital, when, due to regular and healthy deliberate small-portion eating and not drinking alcohol, my weight, in boxers with watch off, dropped from about 115 kg to 107 kg. Needless to say, as soon as I got out of hospital and ate and lived my usual life, it bounced back to 115 kg, where it's been pretty much since I was a young man. The benefit of exercising is that you can eat what you like, when you like, and you needn't worry about watching what you eat, just as long as there is lots of it. I had never known, until recently, the humiliation of realising my favourite pair of jeans no longer fitted me. A 40-inch waist is beckoning.

I imagine we all have a range of our own body weights in our head. There's what we feel we ought to weigh and what we'd like to weigh; then there's 'These scales can't be right' and on up to 'Cripes! I didn't imagine I'd ever weigh that amount'. Now, I know some people do approach a set of scales from the perspective of 'I need to put weight on'. This, however, isn't the problem for most of us, and particularly not for men on the 5–20 lb Zoladex bonus.

Naked and watchless, I get on the brand-new scales an hour or two after Elisabeth and Torsten's *cambriolage* in an Innsbruck car park. There is an immediate choice to be made. Due to technological advance, there is a black switch and the choice is stones and pounds, kilos or just pounds. I wonder, 'Which weighs the least?'

I step on the scales in the privacy of the bathroom, door locked, at 7.30 p.m. on 27 December. 121.7 kg. That can't be right. 19 st. 1 lb. That can't be right either. 267.7 lb. In East Surrey Hospital at the end of June, I had weighed 239 lb.

Because I am tall, when clothed (now in the next size up), I can probably carry an extra 2 st., but at this rate,

I could be 21 st. next June. I could also, if this ache in my shoulder turns out to be not arthritis, be dead by next June. If I want to be buried in St John's, they are going to need a very big forklift truck.

I can't control my PSA, but I can, irrespective of the Zoladex, have some control over my weight. I do have some choice. Is this the same route an anorexic goes down, that they imagine that though they don't have control over parts of their life, they can control their weight, their shape, and gain self-esteem from that dangerous route?

I'll exercise, but I know you can double the amount you do and it won't necessarily affect your weight. If you exercise, unless you want to fall over, you need to eat more. No I'll try to stop the rot by dieting and modest exercising. Like this is original and the rest of mankind isn't reaching the same conclusion as the New Year looms. But I'll start now. In running races or rowing races, often you'll wait for the last lap or going under a bridge before making the final push. I've always found that if you want to win, you should push before the bridge, make an effort just before the last lap. This is just the same: get ahead of the opposition, go before 1 January 2006, Moody Blues it – 'Go now'.

I also know that starting something (in this case it's dieting, but it applies equally to new relationships or new business ventures) is actually the easiest part; making it work is much tougher. The hardest part is ending things well, something I failed to do with Moya. I'll end this diet well at 115 kg and then stay there.

Today is two days since I started. No grazing. Breakfast: a date, peppermint tea with half a spoon of sugar, a mandarin orange, a small slice of bread with a sliver of butter and masses of apricot jam, and a bowl of muesli. Lunch: chicken salad, a small beer (it is still the festive season). Dinner: salad and cold meats, an orange and water. The salad is far nicer than it sounds as it includes potatoes, avocado, carrots, onions, rocket and normal lettuce, and a good olive oil and balsamic vinegar dressing. And cold meats here are a delight.

In East Surrey Hospital, I lost about 2–3 lb overnight and put on 1–2 lb during the day. Here (although I'm saying this after only two days) I seem to lose less overnight but not gain during the day. Is this because I am outside a lot and it is very cold? I'm continuing to weigh myself in stones and pounds, kilos and just pounds.

Friday, 30 December 2005

This morning at 9.00 a.m., I weighed 260.2 lb. Elisabeth has told me that if I don't stop endlessly droning on about my weight, she's going to go back and really put a dent in Torsten's pride and joy. So it's back to money.

Money. OK, first of all, the big money thing: apparently 92 per cent of all human beings live on or below the poverty line; money isn't a big consideration for them, just staying alive is the big thing. I have little idea what their lives are like, they have little idea about ours. So 8 per cent of us are in the privileged position to worry about money. This ranges from the Premiership footballer to the single mum living on a sink estate with three children. The 8 per cent range is from financially enviable to possible financial despair, neither being a place you'd actually want to be (although, on balance, better to be the footballer).

Self-evidently, it would be a good thing if the 8 per cent gave something to the 92 per cent, but it would be an even better thing if the 92 per cent did something for themselves with the encouragement of the 8 per cent. The political process for helping the world to get itself above the breadline has yet to be decided. Maybe Winnie gave us a clue: 'The inherent vice of capitalism is the unequal sharing of blessings; the inherent virtue of socialism is the equal sharing of miseries.'

Money. The little money thing. Although I didn't realise I was doing it at the time, eight years ago, aged fifty, I sort of retired, to live on a small pension and my wits. My Mr Micawber approach to finance has changed over the last six months. Instead of living within my means and hoping something will turn up, as it eventually did for Mr Micawber, who finished up happy in Australia – an axiomatic oxymoron to a Kiwi, but OK with the rest of us. I have developed, since 24 June, a Winnie approach to finance: set your costs and then go find the revenue, and if that doesn't work, sell the family silver.

Saturday, 31 December 2005

This strategy I outlined yesterday is OK, except that periodically, after, say, festivities, celebrations and holiday expenditure, the camel's back of costs is easily broken by an unexpected meeting with a Torsten. The financial spreadsheet doesn't work and gloom can set in. Get over it, Andrew, something will turn up. Anyway, far more interesting things happened today, three things actually, that raised the spirits.

Now, the first two will seem like no big deal and not worthy of comment, particularly if you are a woman or a male who hasn't got locally advanced prostate cancer and isn't six months into monthly Zoladex shots.

First, I went to bed last night about ten and didn't get up until eight this morning, without going to the lavatory. Fantastic. And, as an extra bonus, I woke up with an erection. So it's a pretty good day so far. And then, third, I stood on the scales at 9.00 a.m., again naked and watchless, and there it was: 257.7 lb.

Walking seven miles a day in the mountains and eating as outlined on the 29th seems to work, sort of: 10 lb off, but with no discernable change in my shape. Still, can it get better? It can. It's 31 December, and the New Year is approaching.

Birthdays, Christmas and New Year are days that if I was without a family, I would, I imagine, try to tick off as quickly as possible; but with a family, they can be just the best of days, and today is no exception. Christmas without the fuss and to-do. But New Year and birthdays are just festivals; Christmas and Easter are more significant.

We follow our usual little traditions, although Mouse has had to go back to work, so it's just the four of us and Sophie, who is a daughter of one of Elisabeth's friends and is spending a few days with us. We drink a bit and listen to my choice of music, which is increasingly influenced by Elisabeth and seems to be swinging towards Mahalia Jackson, Peggy Lee, Ray Charles and Luciano, but always includes Van the Man and Randy Newman. A few glasses of almost-champagne, some little smoked salmon things, and even the girls are switching off their iPods, filled with their, to me, alien sounds: Bloc Party, Jimmy Eat World, Elbow, Green Day, Travis, Magic Numbers, Babyshambles, Keane, Goldfrapp, Milo, Franz Ferdinand, the Polyphonic Spree. Are these greyhounds?

We get the fondue going, and over the next couple of hours, we pig out. What diet? It would be a poor fish who couldn't celebrate the Janus moment of 31 December.

At about 11.45 we amble off to stand by the Seekirchl chapel. Seefeld is full. Lots of Russians this year, staying in the smart hotels and – can you believe it – buying jeans (admittedly designer-label ones) selling for, I kid you not,

275 euros a pair. The hotels with that sort of paying guest try to outdo each other with their firework displays. It is spectacular as the colours explode above the snow-covered mountains. We phone Mouse, 'cause 1 January is his birthday. He's at the Royal Oak in Dormansland. We sing happy birthday, the girls go off clubbing and Elisabeth and I go home to sleep. Bye bye, 2005.

Sunday, 1 January 2006

Happy New Year to one and all! I now weigh 260.2 lb. This year, I've decided not to make any resolutions, because the only one of significance would be to do everything I can to be around to see in 1 January 2007. Which would fly in the face of everything I've learned over the last six months, and that is to live in and love and enjoy everything the moment brings, and tomorrow can take care of itself. It's snowing hard.

Friday, 6 January 2006

Epiphany. A new beginning. A significant day in the calendar of the Catholic Church, the day when the three kings, eventually, after trials and travails, by following the star, reached the baby Jesus. Cribs, not in the MTV sense, as in some blinged-up bloke showing you round his tree (actually, as an aside, another US TV programme, *Pimp my Ride*, has a spin-off on German TV called *Pimp mein Fahrrad* – you gotta laugh), anyway, cribs in this snow-covered Alpine landscape now have the three kings added to the manger scene, and they will remain there till 2 February.

All those many years ago, when I had a striped towel over my head and a walk-on part as the third shepherd in Springfield Junior School in Allerton, Liverpool, and after that when I got the same cutting-edge acting role in Westbury Park Primary School, Redland, Bristol, I had imagined the kings got there at the same time as us shepherds. Nope, apparently it was 12 days later.

I seem now to relate everything to and use everything as an allegory for prostate cancer. The shepherds got there early, like their PSAs were under 10, their malignant tumours were contained in the prostate, and they got to have immediate surgery, radical prostatectomies. Most of the shepherds would get lucky. If you have any choice in the matter (and you do), be a shepherd. The kings had PSAs over 10, some well over, and for some the malignant cells had, or maybe had, spread beyond the prostate gland. For them, it was always gonna be hormone treatment and, if appropriate, radiotherapy. The three kings had patience. We kings of the prostate gland must have patience too, and who's to say the longer route isn't the better route? Hey, they were slow but indubitably wise men.

Epiphany follows on in the Christian calendar from Christmas, which is preceded by the four weeks of Advent. Following Epiphany come the forty days of Lent, which precede Easter and Ascension, which is followed by Pentecost, and then it's back to Advent again. See Mum, whatever Mr Hall said, I did pay attention at St Alban's Sunday school. Easter is the big one and is a movable date, as it is based on the lunar calendar and not on some man-made artifice for telling the time or date. The vernal equinox is when the Earth is at right angles to the Sun, which is directly in line with the equator, when the northern hemisphere begins to tilt towards the increasing warmth of Shakespeare's eye of heaven. It happens around 21 March and Easter is the first Sunday after the first full moon after the vernal equinox. For Christians of whatever hue, Easter is the big one. You either believe this stuff or, like my son Mouse, you don't.

Like I believe there are no sharks in Kalamata Bay, because, in part, if I don't believe that, then life will become unbearable. Sure, it may be self-delusion, just to ease the remainder of my life.

And I believe in God. This, too, may be (and is according to Mouse) self-delusion just to ease the remainder of my life. But if you don't believe, then what is the point of anything?

I also believe in myself.

Life, as it does here in this land of spectacular beauty, tumbles one day into another. It's amazing to think the warmth and splendour of being here now has been known to no other generation. As little as maybe 60 years ago, and forever before then, this must have been an area of unmitigated poverty and hardship. Yet here I am, not eating out of choice, and Elisabeth is no better – she deliberately keeps the heating off at night in the bedroom.

For the last few days, I have been living a life of luxury, getting up at about nine, drifting to the breakfast table, which is two steps from the bedroom, about five paces from the lavatory and another five paces in the opposite direction from the sitting room, with the sodding sofa. Having a bowl of muesli, listening to CDs or Radio Tyrol, reading old newspapers, shooting the breeze with Clouds and Stef and Elisabeth and then, about twelve-ish, going for a long walk in the mountains, just breathing, just living, having a bowl of Gulaschsuppe in one of the mountain huts, sitting for an hour or so in the sun, or inside if it's snowing, and getting home about four-ish. Friends and rellies drop by.

Today, Wolfie, the oil man, called to deliver 4,000 l of

heating fuel @ 0.55 euros/l, which is just under 40 p/litre. Seemed cheap to me; maybe there's no tax on heating fuel in Austria. Wolfie, aged 56, is also in the Club. He has an annual medical check. In April 2005, his PSA score had risen to 7, more than double the previous year's reading. He had an immediate biopsy in the Innsbruck Klinik. He had an aggressive Gleason 9. Within a week, he had a radical prostatectomy. They weren't too sure that the tumour was contained. His PSA dropped to negligible levels following the operation, but his latest PSA test, on 28 December 2005, had risen to just under 1 ng/ml. He has some pain in his shoulder, but that could be from heaving oil pipes about all day, or maybe just a touch of arthritis. *Es gibt keine Haifische in Kalamata. Glaubt es, Wolfie.*

Tonight, we are going for cakes and wine with Elisabeth's youngest brother, Georg, who lives next door. He is a plumber, has a smashing girlfriend, a Harley Davidson (so he's a bit suspect) and a company selling waterless urinals. But first I have a date with the scales at 5.00 p.m.

In the last ten days, with a bit of luck, my weight will have dropped from 267.7 lb naked and watchless to X pounds naked and watchless and, of course, after a hot bath. I check in at 254 lb, about 115 kg. I've lost just under 4 oz short of a stone in ten days. And now for cakes and wine next door at Georg's.

Saturday, 7 January 2006

Yesterday lived up to its name. I had a personal epiphany. Do you remember way back on 14 September, when I was a mere two-month apprentice in the interesting new world in which I have found myself (in both senses)? Then, naively but correctly for me, I identified what seemed to me to be the three things you need to deal with if you've got cancer. Which I've copied below.

- **First, the mechanics of your cancer:** at this point in time, the five questions above are my immediate concern.
- **Second, the external factors:** financial position, relationships and other stuff specific to you.
- **Third, the internal factors:** what is going on in your head?

They are, of course, all interlinked, mutually inclusive. Each will sometimes appear to be more relevant than the others; all will change over time as life unfurls.

Well, I now sort of have sort of answers, and here is the revelation, the epiphany: all the answers, for me, were never further away than the next-door neighbour's and often much closer.

First, the mechanics of your cancer: well, my route following my conversation with Mike Swinn in East Surrey Hospital on 24 June has always been to find out more. To talk to as many other men who have or have had prostate cancer as I could find, although not to bother those who prefer to keep their own counsel. I respected their privacy, their choice in dealing with their concerns in their own way. It was none of my business, unless they too wanted to talk about it. My route, always, rightly or wrongly, was to send emails, talk to journalists, keep this record, go on TV, speak at dinners and, most importantly, with my new female side, to actually try to listen to what people said.

I bought some books off Amazon and read them. Dangerous stuff, imagining you know more than you do, but in this instance I think a little knowledge is a good thing, because the cancer is yours, and no one else has a cancer exactly like yours. Listen to yourself.

So, yesterday, I'm deliciously wrecking my diet and talking to Georg's delicious girlfriend, Andrea. It turns out she has just completed her studies at Munich University Medical School, and she is about to do part of her houseman's year in Garmisch, which is half an hour over the border from Seefeld. What has she specialised in? Yep, you're there before I can tell you. Prostate cancer.

Specifically, she has specialised on the quality-of-life issues following radical prostatectomies. She wants to practise her English, I want to know stuff, it's a natural fit. Although I'm careful not to go on, and she is sensitive to both Georg and Elisabeth and also doesn't go on, as she knows their dad died, aged 49, from cancer, as did their mum at 61.

However, I've come a long way since 24 June. I'm now in a room, eating cakes, drinking coffee, talking with my wife, daughter, brother-in-law and brother-in-law's girlfriend about impotence – mine – and incontinence. It all seems pretty easy.

If, say, we run out of sugar, not that I'm using that much nowadays, I'll just pop next door to borrow some and ask my next-door neighbour about why, for example, she thinks some men, when they are having a general medical check-up, refuse to have a DRE.

Be informed. That is, if you want to be informed. If you do, you may find your route is much quicker and easier than you first think.

Second, the external factors: well, first, money. Financially, you should prepare for the worst as soon as possible. Once that is done, move on. If you're bothering to read this, you aren't going to die today. I've adopted the Winnie 'find the revenue to meet the costs' strategy, and it seems to be working. PWC have just asked me to run a pilot Finance for Non-financial Managers course, and Lloyd's Bank have asked me to sit on a panel to judge their managers' presentations. I can do all that.

More importantly, I spent some time trying to find out about how my friends now viewed me and also about myself. Everyone, it seems, not just my friends, appears to take his or her cue from how I/you deal with it all. You're strong, they're strong. Easy, if you can be strong. In any event, you've always got Archibald Cronin's words to keep you happy: 'Worry never robs tomorrow of its sorrow but only saps today of its strength.'

I found myself at some point, if I remember, involved in wallowing about with bad knees in a boat 100 miles off the West African coast with two kind and friendly complete strangers. Good fun, but quite frankly the answer for me was never 100 miles off the West African coast. It was always just across the breakfast table, if I had cared to listen.

Third, the internal factors: this for me has been the strangest part of the experience. If I had ever thought I'd be talking to and having an affair with cancer, that I would speak to her as she would speak to me, then I'd have identified myself as someone who had completely lost the plot. We spoke to each other on 2 December and then again on 22 December. We don't need to speak again. She will not kill me, and she will let the white coats burn out her shadow side sometime this spring, and she will live in me and cause me no harm but give me power.

The bouncy prof will agree to take me off the poison by my next birthday. I will make a full recovery and even keep my prostate intact so I will be able to produce ejaculate and she will be with me. It's gonna be just fine. Stefanos, there are no sharks in Kalamata Bay.

Part Three

Thursday, 21 December 2006

Back in the Austrian tree. Today, now, mid-morning, it is winter bright, Alpine sunny. Bob is on the CD player: 'Spirit on the Water'. There is little snow – global warming, apparently. It was almost a year ago to the day that I spoke to my cancer and she told me how it was going to be, and so it has been. I knew it would be. That's why, on 7 January 2006, I stopped writing. She can kill me, so why should she bother deceiving or lying to me? She loves me. She doesn't see me as the doctor did, Mr 133. No, I'm special, unique, loved, me.

One year on, have I got any advice for you? Well, presumptuous as it sounds, I may have. I mean, please expect no original thought here, lower those expectations. I haven't actually discovered something important that will make a minor contribution to dealing with your life or your problems or your concerns or your issues, whether deep-seated or just those particular testing choices facing you today on life's menu card. I'm afraid you've gotta sort them out by yourself. But I can tell you something, and this is what I can tell you: change your perspective. Then your concerns, issues, secrets will also change. They will become different. Not necessarily better different or worse different. That depends on you – your choice, your call, in your hands. Just different.

Look at you, at your life. The sometimes tedium, the sometimes sense of failure, the sense of frustration or anger or lack of achievement, the sense of things changing, points of reference being removed, stolen or just missing. Come to the conclusion, when you are out there in the blue having a black-dog day, that maybe 97 per cent of your life is rubbish or maybe just even almost rubbish. Well, hang on in there, 'cause that means that 3 per cent is positive, inspirational stuff. And, kiddo, here it is: you gotta live in the 3 per cent, 'cause then it gets a whole lot easier. Self-delusion? Self-deception? Surrendering integrity and reality so you can hide away in cosy land? Maybe. No great depth here. Perhaps all I'm saying is, ignore the big black cloud, just pick up on the teeny-weeny silver lining. Perhaps Eric Idle as the cheery crucifixion victim in *Life of Brian* expressed the same thing much better: 'Always look on the bright side of life.' Now, I couldn't improve on that, but Eric is giving you the what to do; I'm adding on the how. It is perspective, and it is that simple.

Locally advanced cancer was, for me, the catalyst that made me realise that the same thorny crown we all wear from time to time, whatever its guise or form, can become a crown of joy. The blowout in the tyre on the M25 becomes a chance to get to know Elisabeth better and to show her and me I can do stuff and be a roadside hero. The nutter on the bus is actually not a nutter, he is a guy called Hamed whom I can get chatting to.

Here is the really great bit: for you, dear reader, to get to this place, you don't actually need to get locally advanced prostate cancer. It requires only a change in your point of view.

'However, Andrew, easier said than done, particularly if I want that change to have legs.'

Look, it may be simple, but I never actually said it was going to be easy. I had to get a pulmonary embolism, an arrhythmic heart, fall off my bike and bust three ribs and get a PSA score of 133 to get to where I'm now living. All I can do is say how it is for me. You, well, you've gotta sort it out for yourself, 'cause no one else will, and it is simple but not easy.

Thursday, 28 December 2006

Christmas 2006 is now over and gone and was brilliant. One big change from our Anglo-Austrian tradition was that Mouse, Clouds and Stef made Elisabeth and me read the children's Bible story on 24 December. Which we all enjoyed. Revolutionary or what? A shift in power! The old doing what they are told by the young rather than the parents telling their children what to do. Tick tock. I suppose it's the natural order of things and to be encouraged.

I gave Mouse a book on the great philosophers as a Christmas present, 'cause that's the kind of rubbish dad I am. Anyway, yesterday, when he went back via Innsbruck airport hangdoggishly to work, he left the book behind, and I read it, or bits of it. So now I am a total expert on all things philosophical. Last year, Stef gave me a book of short stories about war, and one story, by Elizabeth Bowen, called 'Everybody in London Was in Love', has stayed with me. So equipped with these two pieces of information and the fact that Elisabeth bought a 42-in. plasma screen (it was a real euro bargain, apparently) and Mouse has a stash of DVDs – *Conan the Barbarian*, *Hard Boiled*, etc., you get the drift – including a lot of those ripped-off-from-*The Simpsons* but well written, entertaining, one-linered-up, attention-span-of-a-gnat American cartoon series like *American Dad* or *Family Guy*, I am now, as they say, fully loaded.

In this one particular episode of *Family Guy*, the father (think Homer, but not *The Iliad*) imagines he gets cancer. These cartoons do have edge, so I'm sitting in the room with my kidlets, who are gorgeous and also have edge, and they say nothing but they are fidgety, 'cause the dad is being stoic, just like me. In fact, he's almost using my script: I've had a good life, had my share, intensity of life like never before, etc. Fidget moves on to noticed but unremarked squirm, like when I was 12 in Bristol and I saw a naked African woman on the BBC with my mum in the room. Unremarked, the moment passes, as it did with my mum.

I now know what stoicism is. At least, I think I do. Although not even an articled philosopher with a mere fifteen minutes' study behind him would let you get away with a statement that begins 'I know', because, kid, you don't know anything, at least not for certain. Anyway, like me, or the cartoon dad in *Family Guy*, should you say to someone whose ear you are bending, 'If I die, I've had my share,' then one possible response would be that you were being very philosophical. But maybe you are being, more specifically, stoic, which is a branch of philosophy. Marcus Aurelius (121–180 AD), maybe more of a Roman emperor than a great philosopher, sort of suggests that what happens to us all is the unfurling of providence and that the unfurling of providence is not up to us. Only our reactive attitudes to the unfurling of life are in our gift. So if a dog is tied to a cart, when the cart moves, the dog must go along with it. It can resist, but it will then be dragged uncomfortably along. So the only real choice, for the dog and for us, is to accept our settled fate.

If we are to die from cancer, maybe our only choice is our attitude. Even to a stoic, it is self-evident that that at least is within our domain. Here we have choice. Our attitude is our choice. So here we have absolute control. We may not have control over our cancer, but we can decide on our attitude to our cancer.

Further, and as an added bonus, despite Marcus Aurelius's example, we are not beasts. Maybe, as human beings, we have free will. Maybe, in addition to the ability to control our attitude, we have the ability to bite through the metaphorical rope, with all the attendant risks.

A colony of around 7,000 parakeets roosts every night by the rugby pitch in the Surrey suburb of Esher. This community of birds is probably the result of one parakeet, no, obviously two parakeets flying through the open door of the cage, biting through the rope, or whatever metaphor you care to imagine. No doubt most budgies and parakeets that make that dangerous choice to fly the cage do not survive but succumb to the change of environment or become something else's lunch. As I've just learned, Aristotle, pupil of Plato, pupil of Socrates, espoused, amongst many other things, the mean, the middle course. To the bird in the gilded cage, the mean could be having the untaken option of the open door. Don't fly away to probable death or be locked up with unfulfilled dreams. Take the middle course, be aware of the dangerous option but, crucially, don't take it.

So if our attitude is our choice, then maybe, with all its attendant risks, we should learn as much as we can about our cancer and all the Faustian-pact options to cure, defer or alleviate, but not necessarily take those options. If we do step outside the cage, we may establish a colony of parakeets in Esher or, more probably, we may simply perish.

Me, I'm with Aristotle on this one: open the door but don't fly out. Then again, I am settled and 59. Maybe the imagined immortality associated with youth will see the human race continue to progress and fly. But not for me, not now and certainly not today.

Elizabeth Bowen described London during the autumn air raids in 1940: 'trees on which each vein in each yellow leaf stretched out perfect against the sun . . . birds afloat on the dazzlingly silent lakes . . .' The dead, 'yesterday's living', uncounted and 'the trains and buses in the homegoing rush . . . lighter by at least one passenger'.

> These unknown dead . . . their unknownness . . . could not be mended now . . . So, among the crowds still eating, drinking, working, travelling, halting, there began to be an instinctive movement to break down indifference while there was still time . . . Strangers saying 'Good night, good luck' . . . each hoped not to die that night, still more not to die unknown.

Is it not like this for us with cancer? But for us there is not the immediacy of an air raid or a heart attack, just the corrosion of cancer. We have time, we can enjoy, if we wish, birds afloat on the dazzlingly silent lakes, and each vein in each yellow leaf stretched out perfect against the sun. We can love and be loved, and is this not a wonderful thing?

I'm still with Aristotle, who maintains the good life requires friendship and for whom 'Friends afford the opportunity for goodness and happiness.'

Does not The Prostate Cancer Charity bulletin board, on the Internet in the twenty-first century, give us the opportunity for friendship? We don't know each other, are unlikely ever to see each other and yet, because of prostate cancer, directly or by proxy, are we not now friends?

So, in summary: first, we, if we wish, can determine our

attitude to our cancer. Next, we should learn all we can about our prostate cancer and the treatments and side effects and then, unless we are endlessly brave, choose the mean position. Third, we can enjoy the intensity of life even as both the quantity and quality of that life is diminished. Fourth, and perhaps most important, we can become closer to family and friends, and we can love and be loved.

OK, time to go for a midday-sunshine walk. You can write too much and lose the day, and, as ever, today is the only day of consequence.

Saturday, 30 December 2006

After 51 weeks, I seem to have started writing again, now knowing this may be published. Perhaps it is not just for me. Maybe it is also for you, dear reader, and I'd like that.

I have three thoughts today: a sense of guilt, a need not to apologise and a sense of having something to say. So, like Miss World, in reverse order, here we go.

I've always been highly suspicious of people who believe they have something to say – for example, most politicians – and usually suspicious of what they have to say, too. With people selling stuff and most professional people, like teachers or doctors or estate agents, even if I'm not exactly suspicious – albeit often without any reason – most of the time I'm certainly awkwardly questioning whatever it is they are telling me.

Yet here I am now having the gall to write, imagining I have something to tell you, and yet all I have is my story, which I don't understand, added to a rag-tag of recently gathered information about which I know even less. And the more I learn, the less I seem to understand. This bronze-medal thought is still a work in progress.

Second, in silver-medal position, is a need not to apologise. Many books have, somewhere, a mea culpa, all the mistakes are mine, apologising in particular for repetition, any facts that are wrong, etc., but I feel no such pressure. This is not a factual book on cancer or even an as-yet-unfinished sequential journey from diagnosis to some other point. It is just a jumble, a disconnected stream of consciousness; but you knew that, you're smart, you'd already worked that out. There are no answers here, but there may be, hidden away, something half-developed that gives you something, and I would love that – something, whatever it is, maybe even delivered to your heart.

Finally, gold-medal position, and I have struggled with this thought for some time, in fact since 7 January 2006. It is a sense of guilt, and last night it came crashing home.

Yesterday evening at 6.30 p.m., with Elisabeth and Stef, I went to the Pfarrkirche in Axams, an Alpine farming village on the other side of the River Inn from Seefeld. The Pfarrkirche is a splendid baroque Catholic church that towers above the village as the Hoadl mountain towers above the Pfarrkirche. Agnes Seebacher, aged just 50, died on 26 December 2006 of lung cancer. She was the sister-in-law of Elisabeth's younger sister, Renate. In these villages in the High Tyrol, when someone dies, prayers are said around the body at the same time each day from death to burial, either in the church or chapel or in the home. The Lord's Prayer interspersed with ten Hail Marys in blocks of three.

I met Agnes just twice. She was the youngest, Cinderella daughter, with three elder, reputedly lazy brothers, one of whom had a short marriage, unhappy but blessed with two children, to Elisabeth's sister Renate.

Agnes married her Prince Charming, Peter, when she

was 16 and found love forever. Peter told us, as we stood for a long moment in the ice-dark Alpine light under the high steeple of the Pfarrkirche after the Seelenrosenkranze prayers, that in the autumn, Agnes and he had been mountain-biking up to the Stubai Glacier. She had had no symptoms until late September, and then initially just a barely perceptible breathlessness. A simple X-ray showed a malignant tumour in her lungs as big as a fist, which had spread. It might have been there, growing unnoticed, for five years. No point in surgery, radiotherapy or even chemotherapy. Just palliative care and morphine and eventually a hospice until the cancer had run its course to 26 December 2006.

I have been to three funerals in as many months. Maybe it's just my age.

Carol Holgate lived as long as we have in Dormansland, longer in fact. We were never close friends but she was a good and valued neighbour. She was diagnosed with breast cancer, for the second time, about twelve months ago. We sat near each other in St John's most Sunday mornings, and we shared a weekly look, a glance. We both knew how it was for us. At the packed funeral service a month or so ago, I felt both detached and guilty.

It was a similar feeling to the one I had at Nigel Hook's funeral in Thorveton in Devon. Nigel and I had played rugby together. I was there when his leg broke with a rifle crack and his rugby days were instantly behind him. Our paths crossed often, and he, amongst many, wrote me the kindest of letters when he learned of my diagnosis. Two months ago, he was in France in what would be the middle of nowhere to most but was to him and his French wife their holiday home. He had a heart attack at six and was dead by a quarter past. His funeral was tears and some laughter and a trumpet solo by John Kelly, and then the congregation decamped to the Thorveton Arms and drank too much, and John Kelly and his son Max, both with good voices, sang 'Danny Boy'.

The detachment is easy enough to understand, it's something to do with self-preservation. But the guilt sweeps over me and almost drowns me.

It is eighteen months and one week now since Mr Swinn told me 'It's unequivocal', etc. But who's counting? Well, I am. Each day, I live and love, and I don't count the days to come or look to the future, but I do rejoice as the days grow in number between 25 June 2005 and now. Diane, who posts on The Prostate Cancer Charity bulletin board (her husband Trevor died of prostate cancer in the week before Christmas 2006; the cancer had gone metastatic in 2003), has a saying for all of us on the board: 'Don't count the days, make each day count.'

Why do I feel guilty? Because all around me people have symptoms of cancer, people have dreadful side effects from surgery, radiotherapy, chemotherapy, hormone therapy, there is pain and people die and are dying. Yet I, who seem to have turned into rent-a-gob – who speaks at conferences, writes a book, appears on TV, gives press interviews – I have never had any real symptoms of prostate cancer. For a man of my age, going to the loo once a night is hardly a hardship. I have had, to date, next to no effects from the seven weeks of radiotherapy – mild rectal, bladder and skin irritation for a week or so. The hormone therapy may have temporarily chemically castrated me, but that isn't so bad. My hair is thicker.

Do you know, now, when I go to one of those fund-raising dinner dos for a good cause as a space-filling microcelebrity, when the MC introduces me, instead of a polite round of applause, I now seem to get cheered. I suddenly twigged. I am being cheered because I'm not dead, and, do you know, it's a helluva thing to be cheered for not being dead.

To date, I have felt no pain, yet I see and have seen those whose lives have been truncated or whose quality of life has been diminished. I have experienced none of this yet appear to have stepped into the limelight because I have been diagnosed with locally advanced prostate cancer. My life, as I was heading towards the invisibility of old age, has been given new resonance, and I, quite frankly, enjoy it being resonated. People are endlessly kind to me. Am I just an ageing attention seeker who is milking the benefits while others are paying the price that, so far, I am not? A free rider, centre stage, on cancer? Pass the sick bag, Alice.

Guilt sweeps over me. Never more so than in the ice-dark Alpine light under the high steeple of the Pfarrkirche after the Seelenrosenkranze prayers.

At best, an actor; at worst, something less pleasant.

Sunday, 31 December 2006

There is still no new snowfall. Apparently, ski hire is now non-existent, and the hotel owners are lighting candles in St Oswald's or the Seekirchl or anywhere they can stick a candle. The mind boggles.

I read to Clouds and Stef what I wrote yesterday and listened to what they told me and thought about it overnight, and now, on the eve of 2007, a light has ignited in my head.

Take your own advice, Andrew, and listen to Marcus Aurelius's thoughts cascading down over almost 19 centuries. Sure, it's not easy; but it is simple.

If I go down the path of the hair shirt, self-flagellation, wallowing in guilt and maybe looking for envy in others, who is going to benefit from it? Me? The dead? The living?

If, for the moment, we accept the position of the Stoics, we have choice only over our attitude to the unfolding of providence. Then if misfortune, whatever its form, enters our life, we know we can still have control over our attitude. In this, even if I say so myself, I have so far dealt well with misfortune.

But I didn't listen attentively enough to Eric Idle and probably missed the crucial point the Stoics were making, as they met in the painted porch or colonnade, the *stoa poikile*, in ancient Athens, before Marcus Aurelius gave their thoughts oxygen and legs. Eric actually sang, 'Always look on the bright side of life.' Not 'Look on the bright side of life when you are suffering the slings and arrows' but 'always'. 'Always look on the bright side.' If providence should unfurl to your benefit, you still have control over your attitude. The Stoics had a steadfast indifference to both fortune and misfortune.

So if I should benefit from good fortune (and in my case, at the moment, this is not being dead, feeling no pain and having a good prognosis), my attitude is again in my hands. I can wallow in guilt and the totally unsubstantiated perceptions of others' envy. Or I can take my momentary good fortune and enjoy it. Laugh and be grateful. Be sensitive to others who are less fortunate, but be beholden to no one. Run joyfully with the wind and just be grateful and do good for others. So all I need to do is take my own advice and just change my perspective.

To echo what I said a few paragraphs ago, because I like writing it, I have, so far, dealt well with misfortune, and now, if it is my lot, I must deal equally well with good fortune. When life is 97 per cent great and 3 per cent rubbish, live in the 97 per cent. Perversely, until now,

I have found living in the 3 per cent easier to deal with than living in the 97 per cent. This change in perspective shouldn't actually be too difficult.

I am still only halfway through my treatment and even though *she* has already told me how it will be, I should listen to Diane's aphorism: 'Don't count the days, make each day count.' The date of my next PSA result, 23 April 2007, is out there somewhere, but so too is today, the eve of 2007.

Monday, 1 January 2007

Happy New Year to one and all! I now weigh 260.2 lb. This year, I've decided not to make any resolutions, because the only one of significance would be to do everything I can to be around to see in 1 January 2008. Which would fly in the face of everything I've learned over the last 18 months, and that is to live in and love and enjoy everything the moment brings, and tomorrow can take care of itself. Still no snow.

This is almost word for word what I wrote on New Year's Day last year, except I've had 12 wonderful months, maybe the best year of my lucky and privileged post-war baby-boom life.

Friday, 20 April 2007

It is now almost four months since I last updated this, and before that there was a gap of almost twelve months. It is now, almost to the day, twenty-two months since I was diagnosed with locally advanced prostate cancer. So why am I writing now?

Because next Monday, 23 April 2007, at 3.00 p.m. at the Royal Marsden, Professor Dearnley or one of the other doctors will tell me the result of my PSA sample, taken on 12 April 2007. My last PSA test was six months ago on 23 October 2006 and showed a reading of >0.1 ng/ml. Undetectable – as it has been since my radiotherapy some ten months ago.

The ten months of hormone therapy (one month Casodex 50, ten monthly shots of Zoladex, plus back on Casodex 50 in the tenth month) brought my PSA reading from 133 to 0.13 before the seven weeks of IMRT in May and June of 2006. During the radiotherapy, I continued with the same concurrent hormone treatment, and the cocktail of Casodex and Zoladex has been continued for the last ten months.

So the Prof might say to me on Monday, 'I am delighted to tell you your PSA is still undetectable, we will stop the Zoladex and as a precaution leave you on Casodex 150 mg for another year, with a one-shot dose of radiotherapy to pre-empt possible breast enlargement.' This would mean that no longer would I be chemically castrated. My last one-month Zoladex shot was on 5 April 2007, so by early midsummer my testosterone level should rise. I'd like that.

Alternatively, the Prof might say to me on Monday, 'I have to tell you your PSA has risen.' This could mean that the hormone therapy had gone refractory, stopped having an effect, and the radiotherapy had not burned out the cells the hormones could not get rid of. The white coats would have done their best, but I would be en route to advanced metastatic cancer.

Of course the conversation might be entirely different from either of those suggested above, but I don't think so.

So, three days before this particular conversation at 3.00 p.m. on 23 April 2007 in the AUU of the Royal Marsden Hospital, I'm sort of thinking, well, so far, medically, I've been very lucky. For me, the side effects of the hormone treatment and the radiotherapy have not been dreadful. With the radiotherapy, there was some very short-term bladder, rectal and skin irritation and a little tiredness, but nothing worse than listening to the very dodgy CDs played during the treatment.

With the Zoladex, there came some shallow, mild, infrequent hot flushes, a little loss of muscle, a loss of libido, but that's about it. Also, on the upside, I have thicker hair on my head, less nasal, ear and chest hair and a greater sensitivity to others. I haven't felt particularly tired or emotional and have been able to carry on my life pretty much as before 24 June 2005.

The interesting thing for me is what is going on in my head. The initial change, some 22 months ago, from man without cancer to man with cancer was not easy. Change is always difficult. This is where you were to this is where you are. However, the quicker you adapt to change, the more in control you are, and the more in control you are, the easier it is to learn to live with that change, for you and for others around you.

I remember, in the early days, I decided, 'Don't cross Anxiety Bridge before you need to', and that applies as much today as it did then.

The French scientist Blaise Pascal (1623–62), best known for his experiments with vacuums, has had attributed to him something referred to as Pascal's Wager. His proposition was that the existence or otherwise of God could not be proved by reason and that a wager must therefore be made. Pascal's view was that infinitely more was to be gained by believing in God than by choosing the other side of the coin. How much more frightening would it be to lose the bet if you had chosen not to believe? This, of course, is no proof of the existence of God (you need to go back to St Thomas Aquinas's five propositions, if you want to, for that). No, Pascal is just a man hedging his bets. That's what we guys hanging on the wire awaiting the next marker, which in my case is on Monday, need to do.

If I assume the best of conversations above is the one I will get on Monday, and this is the case, then I'm a happy bunny before and after the Prof's chat. If the Prof tells me stuff I don't really want to hear, then obviously I'm going to be a bit sad post hoc. So, just hedging my bets like any old seventeenth-century French scientist would do, I might as well be happy before the conversation. Self-delusion? Yeah, maybe, but better than crossing Anxiety Bridge. There is always stuff to worry about if you want there to be.

Now, you might say, 'How can you say that, because you might actually feel really ill?' Hang on, when I was diagnosed at 133 ng/ml, I felt great – no symptoms, no pain – but I wasn't great. By the same token, you might not be nearly as bad as you feel.

Then again, a couple of days ago, I had been painting one of our downstairs rooms. Mouse's friend Terry had called round. He was in a T-shirt and had some sort of skin disease on his elbow. The following, hot day, I was walking with Stef when she noticed I had a similar patch of skin disease on my elbow. I scraped at it to no effect, and by the end of the walk I had sunk into a slough of despond, thinking that I'd have to go to the chemist and buy some ointment or whack some more drugs into my already drug-riddled body. Yeah, well, you're there before me: a quick scrub with the scrubbing brush and the paint came off. But I, the guy who is big into Pascal's Wager and other such stuff, had convinced myself I had galloping skin rot. You wanna worry, you can. The pain in my shoulder, which has been there since I was diagnosed: is it bone cancer, but below 1 billion cells so it doesn't register on the bone scan, or is it arthritis? You wanna worry, you can.

However, I've got three days to love life, and that's exactly what I'm going to do. The strange thing is, right now, at this moment in time, I am not actually scared or even worried. In fact, if anything, I am almost excited. This strikes even me as being a little bizarre.

Just before a match or a race, when there is no time to do anything more, the best thing is to try to relax and focus on the event ahead of you. For me, each event, each sport was different. Before a 400-m hurdle race or a 2,000-m indoor-rowing competition, I would be nervous, fearful, the adrenalin would be pumping, a great laxative, and usually I'd feel a need to yawn. I feared those events, as I knew they would hurt. Before rugby matches I never had the same intensity of fear. It was the same when I competed in field events or the 110-m hurdles or sprints, and now in the build-up to veteran rowing races. I think it's because in these sports and events, you never actually cross over into oxygen deficit and the associated pain of hitting the lactate wall. Maximum effort means that unless you condition yourself or run within yourself, normally after about 40 seconds of unrestrained effort you go into muscular oxygen deficit, and if you don't stop, then it hurts – a lot.

On Monday, it is unlikely, as I will just be talking to the Prof, that I will go into muscular oxygen deficit. There will be no physical pain or exertion. Whereas if you told me I had to do a 2,000-m erg race on Monday at max effort, I would now be cacking myself.

So the concern is emotional, in my head, and that, as we know, belongs to me, and I have control. I will not be able to influence the PSA level, but I can stay in control. I can deal with it. Although I still don't understand why

I feel excited. Then again, I don't understand a lot of things. But here's something I now know: for me, it's friends and family and the ordinary things and doing something for other people with no thought of benefit that makes for a happy life. I realise here I am stating a cliché, a platitude, and that if I carry on this way, I'll be looking for if not deification at least some sort of modest halo. Unwarranted. Although I try not to be, I can be lying, deceitful and, like most of us human beings, at times I have feet of absolute clay.

You may have played that game which goes, if you were going to die within a limited time frame, what would you like to do? Now, like many others, I today am actually in this position. Some might concoct a list: whales off New England, see the Victoria Falls, etc. In these last four months, Elisabeth and I celebrated our 30th wedding anniversary in Mauritius, and I went to the Hong Kong Sevens. We are about to visit the gardens at Tresco in the Isles of Scilly. But actually, all I want to do is sit at home with the familiar doing the ordinary, walk Torben and maybe speak at Kidderminster Town Hall or Chesterfield Community Centre to fellow members of the Club. Perhaps I am just getting old. Mauritius was beautiful.

Maybe this is why I am excited: I'm sort of living in limbo land, and on Monday, maybe there will be certainty one way or the other. However, as *she* told me it was going to be OK, I've already decided that it will be OK and I'll start to get my life back as it was. But actually, if it's on offer, do I want it back as it was?

Monday, 23 April 2007

I am a fortunate man. Today, Prof Dearnley, who has always seen me rather than my illness, tells me my PSA blood level has, over the last six months, remained at >0.1 ng/ml. I will not have any more Zoladex injections. As a precaution, I will be kept on Casodex 150 mg per day plus a once-a-week 50 mg tablet of tamoxifen to pre-empt breast enlargement, which is a possible side effect of Casodex. My testosterone will rise as the last monthly shot of Zoladex, given on 5 April, begins to leave my system. The Prof tells me I should come back in three months, on 23 July 2007, when I will have another PSA test and a testosterone test. I am a fortunate man.

Epilogue

Today

So today is every and any day of the rest of my life.

Today in the UK, another 100 men will start on the same journey I started on almost two years ago. Each journey will be different. Each starting point will be different, each treatment and reaction to that treatment will be different. Each one of us has our own unique individual cancer, clumsily defined by where it originates rather than by its very own uniqueness in us. There is no right way to handle the disease. All each of us can say is how it is for him.

I know, for me, there will always be another test, another day when the news will be OK or bad. I know, however, that everybody has issues, concerns, and you just get on with the business of living so long as you have a life to live.

I know all the clichés, aphorisms and platitudes that I have gathered, borrowed, stolen or just made up are amazingly powerful and are things to hang my life on. Cancer is a word not a sentence. Don't count the days, make the days count. Worry never robs tomorrow of its sorrow but only saps today of its strength. There are no sharks in Kalamata Bay.

It seems as if the piece of string has been extended. I appear to have no symptoms or side effects from the seven weeks of IMRT radiotherapy. The Zoladex appears to have cut off my testosterone only for the almost two years during which I was taking it. The testosterone is seeping back. I still have ejaculate. My cancer is still in me, but seems to be causing me no harm. As she told me she wouldn't on 22 December 2005.

So how will I use my gift, given by God with the assistance of the NHS? Well, I will continue to follow Voltaire's advice and cultivate my garden, now knowing that happiness comes from doing things for other people with no thought of financial reward. That is what I'll do. My intentions will be the best. I'll do the right things for the right reasons. I'll do good.

Yesterday, when I was riding my bike in the sunshine on the A22, at the traffic lights in Blindley Heath, a lady car driver pulled out without looking. I braked hard and this time, unlike with Comfort on 8 July 2005, I didn't hit the deck. I yelled a bit, slipped down a gear and throttled off. Then I couldn't help but smile as I adjusted my halo. Had I learned nothing in the last two years? Where is your sensitivity now, Andrew?

Today, I am just another testosterone-filled bloke with road rage. I'm back.

Afterword

In 2006, I asked Andy Ripley if he would speak later that year at The Prostate Cancer Charity's national conference in London. His email shot back like an arrow: 'I'm there or dead,' he said. The response is typical of this giant of a man, a giant physically but more importantly a giant in character, in courage and in determination.

He did speak at that national conference, in the closing session – one of the hardest slots to fill. The audience of nearly 500 people listened intently to his personal story, sometimes in total silence, sometimes in tears, sometimes in laughter. He sent us away totally inspired and encouraged.

Andy has turned his own diagnosis with prostate cancer into something very positive. He has become a great friend of The Prostate Cancer Charity, working with us to raise awareness of what is now the most common cancer in men. We count it a real privilege to include him as such a dynamic force in the UK's growing 'movement for change' in tackling this disease.

John Neate
Chief Executive
The Prostate Cancer Charity

About The Prostate Cancer Charity

Founded in 1996, The Prostate Cancer Charity is the largest voluntary organisation in the UK focused on this disease. Our vision is a world where lives are no longer limited by prostate cancer.

We can best play our part in achieving that vision by aiming to find future solutions through research, while at the same time providing support and information *now* to thousands of the 32,000 men diagnosed every year with prostate cancer and their families, running public-awareness campaigns and lobbying government for improved NHS services.

In its relatively short life, The Prostate Cancer Charity has invested nearly £6 million in research. It plans to make new research grants every year, funding the highest quality research across the UK, on a completely open, competitive basis.

The Charity provides a wide range of information and support on prostate cancer, through its publications, its website (top-ranked by leading search engines) and its confidential helpline – the UK's only nurse-led dedicated prostate-cancer phone line, staffed by specialist nurses.

Much more can be achieved by working together than alone. With that in mind, we strongly emphasise joint work with other charities and professional organisations in getting our message across to politicians and government. The public expect that of us.

Following years of neglect, prostate cancer is at last beginning to receive the attention it deserves. Research investment is increasing, government is paying more attention, political interest is growing and media coverage is stronger than ever. Despite these very positive signs, there is a huge amount of ground to make up, and the support of every section of our community is essential in making the sustained progress we need.

The Prostate Cancer Charity has big plans for the future. It relies entirely on voluntary donations for its income and has no government funding. If you would like further information on how you can support us, please call the Charity on 020 8222 7666 or visit our website, www. prostate-cancer.org.uk.

For further information on prostate cancer, visit our website or call the helpline on 0800 074 8383.

Acknowledgement

The publication of this book has been supported by an unconditional educational grant from the pharmaceutical company sanofi-aventis and a generous donation by Nigel Wray, entrepreneur, businessman and rugby supporter.

The views in this book are entirely those of Andy Ripley and have not been influenced in any way by the book's funders.

Glossary

provided by The Prostate Cancer Charity

Cell cycle: The cycle of activity from when a new cell is produced to its growth and division into further new cells.

DRE (digital rectal examination): the doctor or nurse feels the prostate gland with a gloved and lubricated finger inserted into the back passage (rectum). As well as looking for any abnormalities on the back surface of the prostate, they can also assess the size of the prostate.

Gleason score: scale that shows how aggressive a cancer is by looking at the type of cells in a biopsy sample. The scale runs from 2 to 10, with 2 to 6 being described as non-aggressive, 7 moderately aggressive and 8 to 10 aggressive.

Intensity-modulated radiotherapy (IMRT): a form of external beam radiotherapy. The radiation beam can be adjusted to give different doses to different parts of the area being treated.

Nuclear bone scan: scan of the body, similar to an X-ray, using a radioactive dye to highlight the bones. Shows whether any cancer cells have spread from the prostate to the bone.

Orchidectomy: removal of the testicles, also known as surgical castration. Significantly reduces the amount produced of the male hormone testosterone, which feeds the cancer.

PSA (prostate specific antigen): A kind of protein called an enzyme that is produced by the prostate gland. It is normal to find some PSA in a man's bloodstream.

Pulmonary embolism: a blood clot that clogs up one of the blood vessels supplying the lungs, causing breathing problems and chest pain. Can be fatal.

Trans-rectal ultrasound (TRUS) biopsy: the removal of small samples of tissue from the prostate gland for analysis under a microscope. A small ultrasound probe is inserted into the back passage (rectum). This produces pictures of the prostate and the biopsy needle is then guided into place to take the tissue samples.

Bibliography

Armstrong, Lance, *It's Not About the Bike* (Yellow Jersey Press, London, 2001)

Ballester, Pierre, and Walsh, David, *LA Confidentiel: Les secrets de Lance Armstrong* (La Martinière, Paris, 2004)

Bowen, Elizabeth, 'Everybody in London Was in Love', in *The Vintage Book of War Stories*, ed. Sebastian Faulks and Jörg Hensgen (Vintage, London, 1999); extracted from the novel *The Heat of the Day* (Jonathan Cape, London, 1949)

Foley, Dr Charlotte, 'Chemotherapy for Hormone-Escaped Prostate Cancer – A New Gold Standard', in Prostate Research Campaign UK newsletter, March 2005 (review of I.F. Tannock, R. de Wit, W.R. Berry et al., 'Docetaxel plus Prednisone or Mitoxantrone plus Prednisone for Advanced Prostate Cancer' in the *New England Journal of Medicine*, Vol. 351, No. 15, 2004)

Garfield, Simon, 'Gland on the Run', in the *Observer Magazine*, 8 May 2005

Kimmage, Paul, *Rough Ride* (Yellow Jersey Press, London, 2007)

Kirby, Professor Roger, *The Prostate: Small Gland, Big Problem* (Prostate Research Campaign UK, London, 2000)

Mason, M., and Moffat, L., *Prostate Cancer: The Facts*, OUP, Oxford, 2003

Oesterling, J.E., and Moyad, M.A., *The ABCs of Prostate Cancer* (Madison Books, Lanham, Maryland, 1997)

Parker, S. L., Tong, T., Bolden, S., and Wingo, P.A., 'Cancer statistics, 1996', in *A Cancer Journal for Clinicians*, Vol. 46, No. 1, 1996, pp. 5–27

Soloway, C.T., Soloway, M.S., Kim, S.S., and Kava, B.R. (Department of Urology, University of Miami School of Medicine, Miami, Florida), 'Sexual, Psychological and Dyadic Qualities of the Prostate Cancer "Couple"', in the *British Journal of Urology International* 95, 2005, pp. 780–5